Breakthrough—The True Story
of
Penicillin

Breakthrough

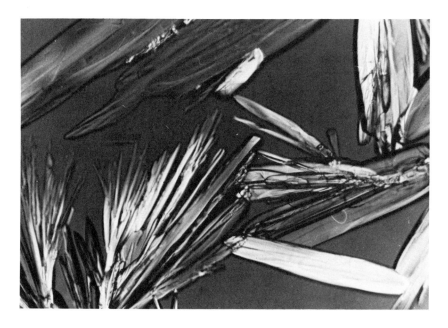

FRANCINE JACOBS

The True Story of Penicillin

ILLUSTRATED WITH PHOTOGRAPHS

DODD, MEAD & COMPANY · NEW YORK

ILLUSTRATIONS COURTESY OF: Abbott Laboratories, 94; Department of The Army, Defense Audio-visual Agency, 115; Sir William Dunn School of Pathology, Oxford, 48, 49, 53, 56, 59, 64, 69, 82, 83, 99; Lady Margaret Florey, 60; Imperial War Museum, 61, 72, 76, 77, 78, 79, 114; St. Mary's Hospital Medical School, Department of Audio Visual Communication, London, 25, 27, 31, 34, 38, 41, 43, 119; Merck & Co., Inc., 2, 14, 107, 112 *top*, 113 *top*; National Archives, 110; Pan American World Airways Photograph, 91; Pfizer Inc., 108, 112 *bottom*, 113 *bottom*; The Royal Society, London, 54; Wellcome Institute Library, London, 20.

FRONTISPIECE: *Penicillin crystals*

2   3   4   5   6   7   8   9   10

Library of Congress Cataloging in Publication Data
Jacobs, Francine.
  Breakthrough: the true story of penicillin.
  Bibliography: p. 123
  Includes index.
  Summary: Describes the history of penicillin from the discovery of the mold by Fleming through the years of work by such scientists as Chain, Heatley, Florey, and Sheehan who purified, tested, synthesized, and eventually presented the "miracle" drug to the world.
  1. Penicillin—History—Juvenile literature.
[1. Penicillin—History]   I. Title.
RS165.P38J33   1985   615'.32923   84-26037
ISBN 0-396-08579-2

For my daughter, LAURIE GAIL JACOBS, M.D.
College of Physicians & Surgeons
Columbia University, May, 1985
With love

ACKNOWLEDGMENTS

THE author wishes to thank the following persons for their help in obtaining photographs for this book:

> Dr. P. N. Cardew, Department of Audio Visual Communication, St. Mary's Hospital Medical School, London, England
>
> J. S. Clark, Administrator, Sir William Dunn School of Pathology, Oxford, England
>
> Eleanor Paradowski, Manager of Communications, Merck & Co., Inc., Rahway, New Jersey
>
> Fred Milesko, Photo Librarian, Pfizer Inc., New York, New York
>
> Thomas A. Craig, Director Media Scientific Relations, Abbott Laboratories, North Chicago, Illinois
>
> William Schupbach, Curator, Iconographic Collections, Wellcome Institute for the History of Medicine, London, England
>
> N. H. Robinson, Librarian, The Royal Society, London, England
>
> Jeffrey Pavey and Allen Williams, Department of Photographs, Imperial War Museum, London, England.

The author also wishes to express her gratitude to Dr. John Whittaker and to Dr. Peter Cook, who went out of their way to make her visit to the Sir William Dunn School of Pathology, Oxford, England, informative and productive.

CONTENTS

Breakthrough—The True Story
of
Penicillin

INTRODUCTION

PICTURE an endless race begun ages ago, and you will begin to understand how science moves forward. Men and women seeking the secrets of nature are the torchbearers in this race. Each carries a bit of knowledge gained through observations and experiments. Science advances as information, like a torch, is passed along from scientist to scientist. Progress stops when promising discoveries are dropped and left by the wayside. It resumes when other scientists come upon the truth, light the torch again, and pass it on.

The development of penicillin was such a race, fraught with obstacles, detours, and surprising turns. It had heroes, heroines, heartbreak, and triumph. Yet, for some forty years, the extraordinary story of the world's first "wonder drug," penicillin, has been hidden in a jumble of misunderstanding and myth. Certain people became famous because of it; others, equally deserving, went almost unrecognized. The remarkable history of this medical marvel, penicillin, however, is stranger and more exciting than the legends about it. This is the true story of what happened and of those who took part in it.

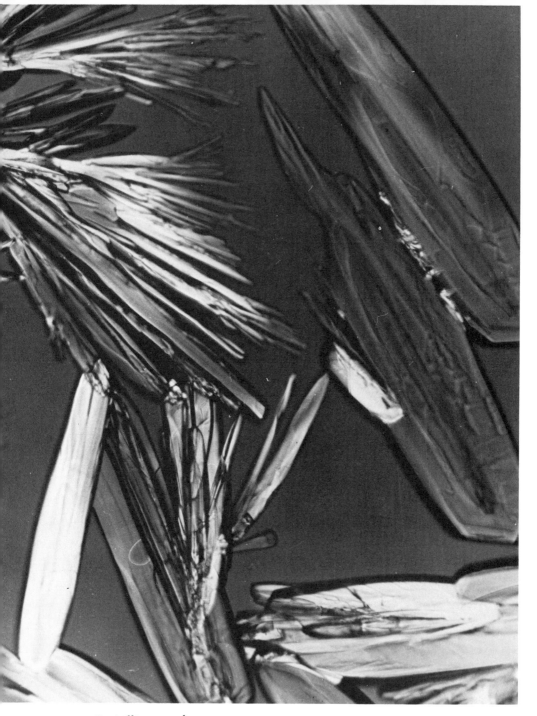

Penicillin crystals

1

EARLY TORCHBEARERS

O N June 26, 1941, in the second year of World War II, two scientists cautiously removed several test tubes from their research laboratory at Oxford University in England. Taking care not to attract attention, they slipped away to a secret airstrip and were whisked aboard an airplane, to begin what was then a hazardous journey to the United States. In a briefcase, they carried the fate of millions of people.

Howard Florey and his assistant, Norman Heatley, were anxious to reach America with their precious test tubes safe. The war was going badly for Britain. She had suffered great losses, and now she stood alone, courageously holding out against the powerful, triumphant forces of Nazi Germany. Britons were forced to endure many sacrifices to defend their island nation. Blockaded at sea by German submarines, Great Britain was plagued by constant shortages of food, medicines, and materials. And funds for scientific research were scarce.

The United States, however, was still at peace. The attack on Pearl Harbor was several months in the future. In the United States, the two Oxford scientists hoped to find help to carry on their work. They would reveal the valuable contents of their briefcase to the Americans. They would share their test tubes of blue-green mold, fungus that looked like any ordinary, common mold found on stale bread or rotting fruit. But this particular mold they were bringing to the United States was very special. It produced a remarkable yellow substance called penicillin.

The story of penicillin really begins approximately 140 years before Howard Florey and Norman Heatley undertook their wartime mission to America. At that time, about 1800, outbreaks and epidemics of plague, cholera, typhoid, tuberculosis, scarlet fever, and other dread diseases continued to ravage populations as they had for centuries. Medical science had progressed little in two thousand years. Primitive treatments like driving out demons from the ill, wearing garlic or magic charms, using smelly oils and hot packs, baths, bloodletting, and much other hocus-pocus persisted. Treatments were sometimes as horrible as the illnesses they were supposed to cure. Theories about what caused plagues and epidemics abounded, but all of them were wrong.

Then, in 1796, Edward Jenner, a country doctor in England, found a way to prevent smallpox. In Jenner's time, the average life-span for everyone, from birth to death, was only thirty-one years. And one out of every ten children under the age of four died from smallpox. Jenner observed that dairymaids who suffered a mild infection called cowpox seemed to be protected from the dread smallpox. So the wise country doctor inoculated other people, infecting them with cowpox pus, and found that it was possible to give them the same protection, or immunity, that the dairymaids had.

Jenner, in his lifetime, never learned what caused smallpox (a virus too small to be seen under an ordinary microscope) or why his procedure worked (it stimulated the body to produce antibodies, a defense against disease). Nevertheless, Jenner's remarkable discovery lit a torch that led medicine out of darkness and superstition and helped to turn it into a science.

Some thirty years after Jenner's death, in the 1850s, a bold French chemist, Louis Pasteur, became interested in the microscopic organisms called bacteria, or germs, that were spoiling the production of wine. Pasteur's work led to a method of controlling the growth of bacteria. This technique, which dairymen also put to use to protect milk from souring, became known as "pasteurization." Pasteur continued to study bacteria and, in 1870, discovered that germs were causing a disease in silkworms that was ruining France's silk industry.

In solving this problem, Pasteur hit upon a momentous truth: microscopic organisms could cause disease. Through the ages, some few scientists had guessed that tiny, living organisms, too small for the naked eye to see, might cause disease. But they were scoffed at and disregarded. Now, at last, Pasteur had proven this to be true.

Pasteur's brilliance was such that his mind could leap quickly from small experiments to great theories. He wondered, if germs could make silkworms ill, might they not also cause other diseases, even diseases in people? The question he considered rapidly gave birth to the notion that human illnesses might well be caused by harmful bacteria. Pasteur became even more fascinated by germs now. His experiments showed that microscopic organisms were all around— in air, dust, and water. Eager to tell the world about germs, Pasteur proclaimed his "germ theory of disease" and excited medical scientists everywhere.

In Scotland, a respected surgeon, Joseph Lister, became interested in Pasteur's germs. If Pasteur was correct and germs were everywhere, Lister reasoned, then they must be getting into surgical wounds. Perhaps germs caused the pus, swelling, and fevers so many of his patients developed after surgery. Despite Lister's best efforts, two out of five people died of infections following successful operations.

So Lister began searching for ways to protect his patients from germs. He found a chemical, carbolic acid, that was used to treat sewage, and he prepared mild solutions of it. He washed his hands and instruments and soaked bandages and dressings with the chemical to kill germs. He applied it to wounds and sprayed it in the air during operations. His method soon produced impressive results. No longer were so many patients surviving surgery only to die during recovery from germ-caused infections, sepsis. Lister's practice of killing germs to prevent sepsis was to become standard procedure in surgery everywhere. He was the first physician to use chemicals to prevent infection; these agents became known as antiseptics. Lister had taken a light from Pasteur's torch and carried it in a new direction.

Meanwhile, in Germany, a brilliant, methodical physician, Robert Koch, had also begun to investigate the role bacteria played in disease; he laid down important guidelines that other scientists would follow. In 1876, Koch found the germ responsible for the deadly disease anthrax, which affected cattle, sheep, goats—and, sometimes, people. For the first time ever, a scientist had shown that a specific germ could not only produce a disease in animals but also in human beings. In 1882, Koch discovered another germ to be the cause of the dread "white plague," tuberculosis. The race to identify germs that caused diseases became worldwide. Bacteriology, the study of germs, had come of age in medicine.

And Pasteur was busy during this time also. He too worked on anthrax and on another animal disease, chicken cholera. Pasteur was a shrewd observer, and he was familiar with the work of Jenner. Perhaps it was the light of Jenner's torch still aglow in Pasteur's mind that caused him to recognize, one day, the meaning of a minor experimental incident. Pasteur, intending to infect chickens with cholera germs, unintentionally had used an old culture of the bacteria, causing the birds to develop only a mild case of cholera. When he reinfected these birds with strong, fresh cholera germs, the chickens remained well. They seemed to be protected. Surprised by this result, Pasteur must have been struck by the similarity of this accident to Jenner's work with cowpox to prevent smallpox. Could old, weakened germs, he wondered, be used to protect animals and people against harmful infections?

Now almost sixty, Pasteur energetically threw himself into testing his new idea. But Pasteur was not a physician, so he was forced to confine his efforts to animal diseases. He returned to his earlier work on anthrax and produced a mixture of dead and weakened anthrax germs that successfully protected animals against anthrax. Pasteur called this material a "vaccine." He named it that deliberately to honor the memory of Jenner. For "vacca" in Latin means cow. And so this method of giving protection, or immunity, against disease became known as "vaccination."

Pasteur next developed a vaccine for rabies, a disease that affected dogs and other animals, making them vicious. People were terrified of rabies. With good reason. For anyone unfortunate enough to be bitten by a rabid animal suffered a horrible fate. The disease attacked the brain, causing victims to behave like mad dogs. They frothed at the mouth, were dangerous to control, and—in the end—they always died. So, when word of Pasteur's vaccine for rabies spread, it brought desperate pleas for help from people who had been bitten. Pasteur, however, lacking a medical degree, dared not experiment on human beings with his vaccine.

On July 6, 1885, however, in an act of extraordinary courage, putting his whole career at risk, Pasteur injected nine-year-old Joseph Meister, who had been attacked by a rabid dog. The boy lived. Young Meister was the first person ever to survive rabies. Naturally, this case added greatly to Pasteur's prestige and dramatically called the world's attention to the promise of vaccines.

Soon laboratories in many countries were working to develop vaccines.

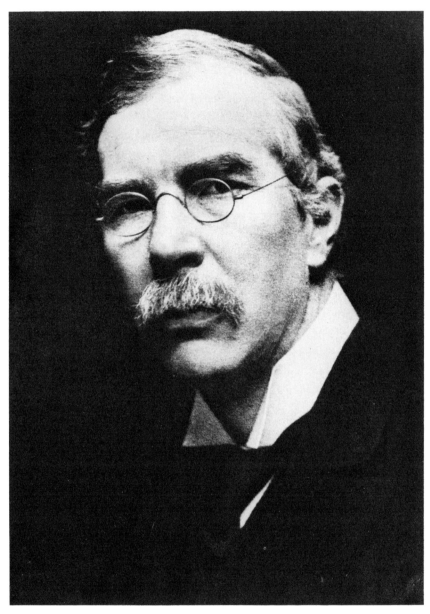

Sir Almroth Wright, developer of the typhoid vaccine, who predicted that immunology would be at the forefront of modern medicine

2

THE INOCULATION DEPARTMENT

IN 1893, in England, a powerful and influential physician, Almroth Wright, eagerly entered the race to develop vaccines. Wright was working with bacteria at the British Army Medical School. The disease that interested him most was typhoid, a sickness caused by a small, rod-shaped germ. The typhoid germ is carried by contaminated water, milk, or food and is always a threat wherever unsanitary conditions exist. It is a deadly disease, killing 10 to 30 percent of its victims after a short, miserable illness with chills, fever, aches, and diarrhea. It is a particular threat to soldiers at war because they often are forced to camp in the field, where sanitation is frequently makeshift and poor.

It took Wright six years to make an effective vaccine to prevent typhoid. Wright was certain that his vaccine could save many lives. So he wanted every British soldier to be inoculated with it before leaving for South Africa to fight the Dutch settlers in the Boer War (1899–1902). But Wright could not convince army authorities to order this, and only those men who volunteered to receive the vaccine were inoculated. As a result, thousands of troops who might have been spared needlessly suffered typhoid. In fact, more British soldiers died from this disease than from the fighting in South Africa.

Outraged by this foolish waste of life, Wright resigned his position at the British Army Medical School in 1902 and joined the faculty of St. Mary's Hospital in London. There he created a department to study germs, vaccines, and immunity. Wright was a huge, impressive man who enjoyed authority and being Chief of his own department. He was very demanding of himself and of his staff. But there was another side to him, also. To his patients, Wright was a gentle, caring physician anxious to relieve their suffering. And he was convinced that the best way to fight diseases was to prevent them by protecting people with vaccines.

Vaccines became the medical wonders of the early 1900s. The new science that used vaccines to protect, or immunize, against infectious diseases—diseases caused and spread by microscopic organisms— was called Immunology. It was the most exciting field of medicine at that time. In a few short years, immunologists had produced vaccines to protect against some of the greatest enemies of humanity: plague, cholera, typhoid, and typhus. Typhus is a disease different from typhoid. It produces fever, headache, and red spots. Typhus, caused by microscopic organisms tinier even than bacteria, is transmitted by the bite of an infected flea.

But still no effective vaccines were found for many diseases. The germs causing tuberculosis, scarlet fever, meningitis, pneumonia, and other infectious diseases went on crippling and killing adults and children. Infections still killed more people than all other causes of death combined. While vaccines had been made to prevent certain diseases, medicine had few weapons with which to fight infections once they struck. Doctors tried to comfort their patients but they could not cure them; they often were forced to sit helplessly by a patient's bedside with little to offer but hope.

Chemical antiseptics were already widely used to kill germs outside the body and in open wounds, but they were too harsh to be taken internally. Few medicines existed that could be swallowed or injected safely to fight infections. There was quinine from the bark of a South American tree to treat the infectious tropical disease called malaria, which causes high fevers and teeth-chattering chills. It is spread by the bite of certain mosquitoes. Another medicine in use was the chemical mercury. It was given to sufferers of syphilis, an infection that can paralyze, blind, and cause insanity. But mercury was highly dangerous. Patients who took it risked damage to their kidneys and the loss of their teeth.

Scientists had yet to learn how to make medicines from chemicals in the laboratory that could fight infectious diseases inside the body. About 1900, in Frankfort, Germany, the chemical dye industry was growing rapidly. Here scientists were creating colorful new dyes by combining chemicals. This activity attracted a German friend of Almroth Wright, a physician-chemist, Paul Ehrlich. Ehrlich had worked in Robert Koch's laboratory and well understood the role germs play in disease. He believed that a drug might be made from chemicals that could cure infections. So Ehrlich sought a chemical that would act like a "magic bullet" to kill a specific disease germ.

A lively, likeable man who puffed away on cigars and enjoyed a funny story—especially if he told it—Ehrlich searched among the dyes, seeking his cure. He worked for five years without success. Finally, still convinced he would find it, Ehrlich turned from the dyes and began to test other chemicals. He started to work with compounds of the element arsenic and persevered three more years. Success finally came with the 606th compound he tested. This chemical killed the spiral-shaped germ that caused syphilis; it cured laboratory animals infected with the disease. Ehrlich called his "magic bullet" Salvarsan (from the Greek, meaning saved by arsenic) or, simply, "606."

Salvarsan was soon successfully tested on human patients with syphilis. Ehrlich's "magic bullet" lifted a new torch and raised the hopes of physicians everywhere. For the first time ever, a scientist had shown that a drug could be developed purely from chemicals to fight infection. Chemotherapy, the use of laboratory-made drugs to cure disease, was born. So about the turn of the century, from 1890 to 1910, within the short space of some twenty years, immunology and then chemotherapy arose to change the future direction of medical science.

Ehrlich brought samples of Salvarsan to his good friend Almroth Wright—now Sir Almroth Wright—whose achievements in producing the typhoid vaccine had led to knighthood, an honor awarded to him by King Edward VII of England. But the famous doctor was doubtful about chemotherapy. He feared that drugs might only treat the symptoms, not the causes, of disease, and he continued to favor immunology. In the long run, he believed, vaccines that enabled people to resist diseases would prove to be more valuable than drugs. "The doctor of the future," he predicted, "will be an immunizer."

Wright chose bright young scientists from around the world to work in his laboratory. One such research worker was a short, broad-shouldered, 29-year-old Scot named Alexander Fleming. Fleming was a quiet, soft-spoken physician who said little but was admired for being a keen observer. "Flem," as he was sometimes called, also had nimble fingers. Probably his reputation for sure-handedness prompted Wright to assign Fleming the duty of preparing Salvarsan solutions and giving the drug to syphilitic patients at St. Mary's Hospital. For it was necessary to inject Salvarsan with care directly into the patient's veins so that the fluid passed into the bloodstream without irritating surrounding tissues.

At this time, 1910, injecting anything directly into a vein was still new and dangerous. Fleming, with his agile hands, became expert at giving Salvarsan, and he was probably the first physician in Britain to use the new drug. But Fleming shared Wright's view that drugs probably were not the answer to treating infectious disease. He made

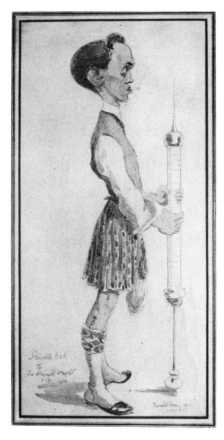

"Private 606." This cartoon of Alexander Fleming by his friend Ronald Gray shows the doctor in 1911, in the kilts of his Scottish regiment, holding a hypodermic syringe instead of a rifle.

an exception for Salvarsan, however, when he observed how fast it cleared up the ugly sores of syphilis.

Fleming added to the small salary he earned as a researcher by maintaining a private medical practice. In his long white physician's coat, and always with a tidy bow tie in place, the kindly Fleming easily won the confidence of worried patients. He also injected the harsh, yellow Salvarsan solution with such skill that other patients soon flocked to his office, and he prospered. Members of the London Scottish army regiment to which he belonged joked about this. His buddies nicknamed him "Private 606."

Wright's department where Fleming worked was growing in size and importance. From two cramped rooms, which shook from trains chugging through tunnels beneath the hospital, the department moved to a round, brick tower in the southeast corner, the Clarence Wing. It was now officially called the "Inoculation Department." The department faced onto Praed Street, the main thoroughfare to London's huge Paddington Station nearby. Outside, a steady stream of horse-drawn buses and cabs made their way along Praed Street, passing dusty junk shops and the local pub, or tavern, where Fleming and his colleagues sometimes enjoyed a half-pint of bitters (ale).

There were four floors to the tower that housed the Inoculation Department. On each level, a small ward meant for six or seven patients had been converted to offices and laboratories. But these too soon became cramped and overcrowded, forcing Fleming at times to juggle his equipment and rearrange his experiments. Even Wright didn't have a place of his own. White-tiled laboratory tables were cluttered with microscopes, slides, racks of test tubes, Bunsen burners, incubators, and petri dishes, those small, round, flat glass cases in which bacteria are grown. The place had a smell, too; it came from a simmering pot of hot oil used to sterilize syringes.

Fleming and his group had several duties at St. Mary's. Wright insisted that his researchers keep contact with patients. So on a typical day, Fleming spent his morning visiting and examining patients in the hospital's wards. When these rounds were done, he saw outpatients. A mass of poor, ailing people regularly waited each afternoon in the stairway leading to two wards in the Inoculation Department, hoping for a treatment that might cure their painful ulcers, boils, or festering sores. Fleming took samples of their blood and pus and used them to develop vaccines. The department also produced vaccines for sale to the largest of the few pharmaceutical companies that existed at that time; this provided income to help pay its expenses.

It was usually late afternoon before Fleming was able to get to his

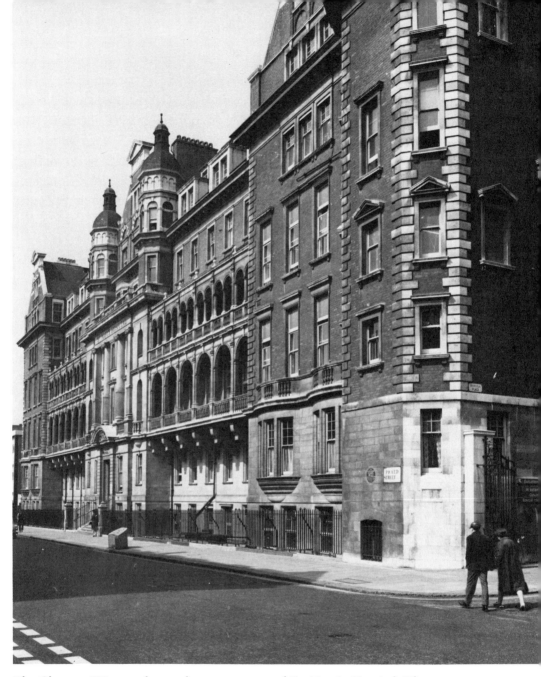

The Clarence Wing at the southeastern corner of St. Mary's Hospital. The third floor up, with three windows across the right-hand corner of the building, housed the laboratory where Alexander Fleming discovered penicillin.

laboratory bench. There he carefully transferred the patients' specimens to test tubes and petri dishes containing agar, a gelatin made from seaweed that is an excellent medium for growing germs. He then placed these cultures of germs in incubators to grow. From these and similar cultures, Fleming prepared microscope slides to identify the germs, and he prepared vaccines. This work demanded much skill. And it was dangerous. Two members of Fleming's group died of infections they got while performing it.

Fleming enjoyed his work. If the long hours or crowding bothered him, it never showed. He did not complain. Fleming made much of the equipment he used himself. He stretched tubes of glass in the flame of a Bunsen burner, drawing them out into needle-thin straws, pipettes. These he used to transfer small quantities of fluid from one vessel to another. In his spare moments, Fleming enjoyed making little animals from leftover glass; he gathered a sizeable collection.

In the evenings after dinner, when their regular duties were done, the research group would meet to discuss their work with Wright. They often gathered over tea in a little room at the top of the stairs they called the library, though it had no books. These discussions sometimes lasted well into the night. Fleming was a valued member of the group. He had a knack for solving problems and could think up just the right experiment to prove a point. Despite his good standing among the group, however, Fleming spoke little at these meetings. He was a person of very few words and did not discuss his ideas or show his feelings easily. These personality traits were to handicap him later.

3

A VALUABLE LESSON

THE same events that influence the lives of ordinary people also affect the course of science. Political changes, economic times, natural disasters—and wars—can slow or quicken the progress of science. World War I (1914–1918) brought advanced new weapons: military airplanes, submarines, armored tanks, and poison gas. And high-explosives, introduced for the first time in bombs and artillery shells, caused casualties on a scale never seen before. Shrapnel, metal fragments from bombs and shells, tore through soldiers' uniforms and into their flesh. These dirty, twisted bits of metal carried soil bacteria and produced horrible infections: tetanus, or lockjaw, a usually fatal disease that tightened, or locked, the victim's muscles; and gas gangrene, a deadly disease that made wounds bloat and poisoned the blood. As the number of wounded mounted, surgeons in the field called upon scientists for help.

England entered the war in August, 1914. She came to the defense of Belgium, which Germany had invaded in order to attack France. Two months later, in October,

Sir Almroth Wright, now a Lieutenant-Colonel, and members of the Inoculation Department were on their way to France. The British army had taken over a recreation center in Boulogne on the west coast of France and turned it into a hospital. Alexander Fleming, a Lieutenant in the group, helped set up a research laboratory in the building's attic where a fencing club used to practice. Their mission was to study wound infections and develop better ways to treat them.

The wards below were crowded with wounded; men with shattered limbs, damaged bones, and torn muscles, nerves, and blood vessels lay on camp beds and stretchers in pain. Many were out of their minds with high fevers caused by infections. The surgeons did what they could to save lives. Frequently this meant amputating infected arms and legs. But even these extreme measures often failed to stop the germs from spreading. Infections took a terrible toll.

The standard treatment for infections in the first World War was to open battlefield wounds and pack bandages soaked in antiseptics into them. As these antiseptic packs became sodden with pus and fluid, nurses replaced them with fresh dressings. Alexander Fleming doubted the value of this treatment. He was convinced that, though the harsh antiseptics killed germs, they did more harm than good. Some thirty years earlier, the Russian biologist Elie Metchnikoff had shown that white blood cells are an important natural defense against infection. They attack and destroy invading germs. Fleming believed that antiseptics interfered with this natural defense. He also felt that these strong chemicals were ineffective in cleansing wounds.

Fleming devised an experiment to prove his point. He melted the bottom of a test tube and drew the glass out into hollow points to resemble a jagged wound. Then he poured in infected blood serum, the clear fluid free from red blood cells that oozes from cuts and wounds. The serum spread over the rough edges of the "wound." Now he rinsed the model with strong antiseptics. But no matter which

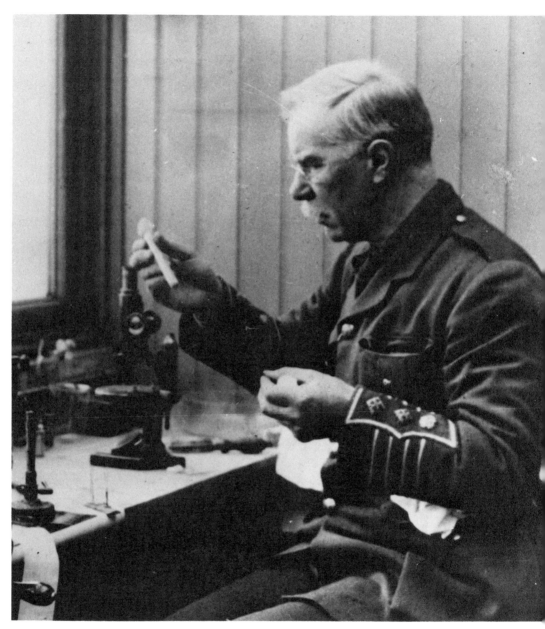

Sir Almroth Wright with the British Army in France during World War I

antiseptic he used, each time he put clean, fresh blood serum into the test tube, the serum became infected. The antiseptics had killed many germs, but some bacteria, hidden in the jagged edges of the "wound," always remained to grow again. The experiment showed that antiseptics failed to clean infected wounds.

But what to do? Fleming and Wright suggested that the routine use of harsh antiseptics be stopped. They advised that only gentle cleansing solutions be used and that the surgeons concentrate their efforts instead on removing all dead and dying tissues from the wound; the damaged tissues gave germs a place to hide and thrive. But Fleming and Wright found surgeons reluctant to change their ways. It was discouraging to recognize the truth and be unable to convince others. Slowly, however, Fleming and Wright did persuade many field surgeons to drop harmful methods and adopt more helpful ones.

This wartime experience with antiseptics strengthened Fleming's belief that chemicals would not play an important role in treating infectious disease. Indeed, except for Ehrlich's Salvarsan, scientists had been unable to find other "magic bullets." Chemotherapy, which had once seemed so promising in the battle against disease, had almost come to a standstill. Infections still took the lives of wounded soldiers, while pneumonia and other diseases killed countless other men, women, and children. Pneumonia, an infection of the lungs, killed one out of every three of its vicims, and it was third among the leading causes of death in the United States at that time. Scarlet fever, diphtheria, meningitis, and other bacterial diseases claimed thousands of additional lives. Infectious diseases caused half the deaths of all children under six years of age. And infection continued to be a constant threat in childbirth and surgery.

This is where medicine stood in the western world when World War I ended. Eight-and-one-half million lives had been lost in the war, but peace did not end the dying.

In 1918–1919, a great epidemic, a spread of infectious influenza, swept through whole populations in Europe and crossed the Atlantic Ocean to America. Influenza, caused by a virus, attacked peoples' lungs, making it hard for them to breathe. The disease often led to infection of the weakened lungs by bacteria. The influenza epidemic killed more than twice the number of people that died in the fighting of World War I.

In January, 1919, Wright and Fleming returned to the Inoculation Department at St. Mary's Hospital in London to resume their work. Fleming came back a married man. While on leave during the war, he had wed Sarah Marion McElroy. The new Mrs. Fleming was a nurse and the successful owner of a private nursing home in London. Her income from the sale of this establishment enabled Fleming to give up his private practice and spend more time at St. Mary's. There, as a member of the medical college faculty, he began to teach. But his reserved manner made him a poor lecturer. Medical students complained of difficulty in hearing him, and they found his classes boring. Fleming's old handicap in presenting his ideas and communicating effectively continued to plague him.

In 1921, Fleming became Assistant Director of the Inoculation Department. He moved into a tiny laboratory of his own in the round brick tower near the staircase. It was a dingy little room lined with bookcases and dark cabinets. Even here, Fleming had to share space with other members of the group. His well-stained workbench, however, faced the window overlooking Praed Street. A smiling photograph of the Russian Metchnikoff, in full beard, failed to soften the dreariness of the place.

Though Fleming was careful and well organized, he was not particularly tidy. There was a striking difference between his table, cluttered with stacks of petri dishes containing old cultures, and that of the group's new member, Doctor V. D. Allison. And Fleming teased the younger man about this. One day, late in 1921, Fleming looked at his messy work space and decided to clean up the pile of old

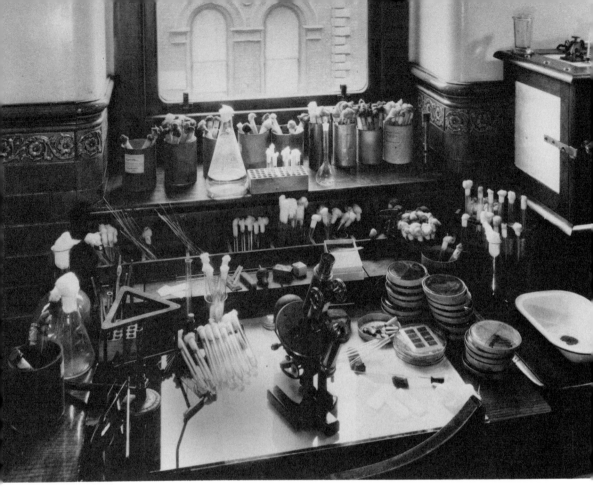

Fleming's laboratory at St. Mary's Hospital. Photo was taken in 1928.

cultures lying there. But he was the kind of person who could not throw anything away easily. So he examined each petri dish carefully before discarding it. While doing this, he noticed something curious. On one plate, unwanted germs had gotten in to establish large, yellow colonies. These had overgrown the surface of the plate like weeds in an untended garden. But something was killing the invaders. The plate had clear spaces, free of germs.

Fleming tried to remember the history of this peculiar petri dish. In it he had prepared a culture of mucus taken from his running nose on a day when he had a cold. Germs from the air had obviously settled on the surface of the agar plate and grown there, too. But something—perhaps something in his mucus—was dissolving the germs that had come from the air and landed in the plate.

Fleming found the airborne intruders, the "weed" germs, to be a new, but harmless, variety of bacteria. He grew them in a test tube of broth, and the germs made the broth cloudy. Now to test his idea about the mucus, Fleming added some to the broth. The cloudiness in the test tube vanished. The germs dissolved.

Fleming got Dr. Allison to help him determine what in his nasal mucus had dissolved the germs. They tested to see if other body secretions might also contain the mysterious germ-killing substance. They found that it was also in tears. They squeezed lemon juice into their eyes to make tears. But they needed more. So laboratory helpers cried for them also and were paid for their tears, each according to the amount he supplied.

The mysterious germ-killer turned up also in saliva, hair, nails, skin, and, in fact, in all tissues. It was highly concentrated in egg white and also present in flowers and other plants. Fleming guessed it would prove to be an enzyme, a natural substance that brings about chemical changes. So when the research group discussed Fleming's discovery, Wright named it lysozyme. ("Lyso" from the Greek word *lysis,* meaning to dissolve, and "zyme," the Greek word meaning to mix).

By accident, but not merely by chance—for he was a keen observer and was eager to experiment—Fleming had discovered a natural antiseptic in the human body itself.

Excited with his new find, Fleming eagerly presented a scientific paper on lysozyme before the respected members of London's Medical Research Club in December, 1921. The evening, however, was a disaster. Fleming's dull style of speaking undid him. His audience listened patiently, but when he finished, no one bothered to ask a single question. Instead, there was a humiliating silence. Fleming, stung by this cool reception, left the meeting stubbornly determined to continue his research on lysozyme. He did not accept the judgment of the club members that the work was unimportant because lysozyme was effective only against harmless germs.

Fleming put six more years of effort into lysozyme and published six more scientific papers on it. But his hopes were never realized. The substance never proved useful in treating infectious diseases. Nor was he ever able to purify it. Neither he nor the other members of the Inoculation Department were trained chemists. Finally, in 1927, Fleming's interest turned from lysozyme to other projects. Although lysozyme was never to play an important role in the fight against disease, it would prove to be a valuable lesson.

4

DISCOVERY—AND DISAPPOINTMENT

TEN years had passed since the Great War ended, and the world outside the Inoculation Department at St. Mary's Hospital was in turmoil once more. It was 1928. The economies of Germany and other European countries had collapsed, unemployment was rising in Britain, and the financial markets were shaky. In America, people were laughing at the first Mickey Mouse movie, and Herbert Hoover was campaigning to become President.

Progress in chemotherapy for infectious diseases had almost come to a halt. Since Salvarsan, eighteen years earlier, the only advance had been a drug for African sleeping sickness developed by the German company, Bayer. Still nothing existed to treat pneumonia and other major infections.

One day early in September, Alexander Fleming, now a full professor of bacteriology, returned to St. Mary's from his summer cottage in the country. Fleming was forty-seven. Though he no doubt had enjoyed his vacation, gardening, fishing, and relaxing with his wife and

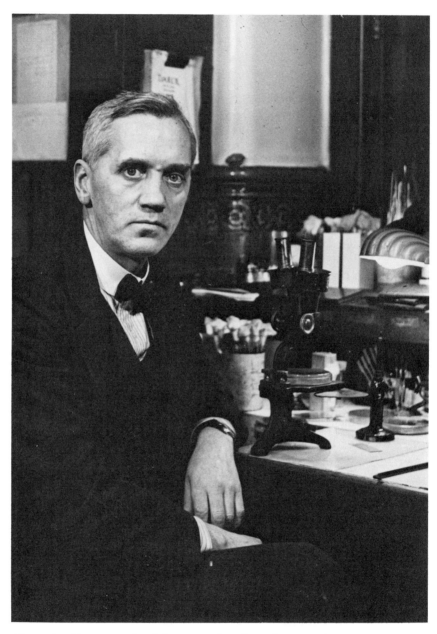

Alexander Fleming at his laboratory bench in the Inoculation Department of St. Mary's Hospital about the time he discovered penicillin, 1928

four-year-old son, he was probably eager, after weeks away, to get back to his research.

First to clean up the clutter of cultures Fleming had once again left piled on his laboratory bench. He had been studying staphylococci, pus-producing bacteria common on the skin that look like bunches of grapes under a microscope. The germs had come from the hospital clinic, from patients with boils. As was his habit, Fleming examined each culture plate before discarding it. While he was doing this, a former assistant stopped by, and the two men joked about the untidy mess. The neglected cultures were old and useless. There, for example, on top of a stack of discarded plates was a petri dish with mold growing in it.

Molds are simple, non-flowering plants that belong to the family called fungi. They form minute reproductive bodies, known as spores, that float about in the air and often find their way into bacterial cultures and grow there. Every time a researcher lifts the cover of a petri dish to deposit or remove the germs he is growing, he risks mold spores getting in and contaminating the culture. Fleming's plate, a culture of staphylococci, had been lying around for weeks, ample time for a mold to grow.

Fleming was suddenly interested in the ruined plate. Around the blob of mold, a wide, clear area had formed from which the staphylococci had disappeared. And beyond this clear zone, other colonies of staphylococci were dissolving. The yellow colonies were beginning to resemble drops of water.

Perhaps someone else, less knowledgeable, would have dismissed this incidental finding as merely one of those freakish mishaps that often occurs during research, an interesting, but unimportant, accident leading nowhere. Major developments in science, the breakthroughs that win prizes and make headlines, almost never result from fortunate accidents. The great Pasteur himself scoffed at luck. Fate, he maintained, only helps those who are prepared to make the most of it.

39

But fortune, which had teased Fleming before with lysozyme, now tested him once more. Fleming instantly saw the similarity to his earlier discovery. But this time, something, perhaps something from the mold, was killing *harmful* germs. The usually calm and even-tempered Scot was excited.

Fleming was eager to tell others in the department about his discovery. He took the plate into the main research laboratory and showed it there. Then he took it downstairs to C. J. La Touche, the group's expert on molds. He could hardly wait for Wright to come in that afternoon so he could show it to him. But no one, not even Wright, was impressed. Fleming's earlier discovery, lysozyme, had cost years of effort that only ended in disappointment. Its ghost still haunted the department. His colleagues were kind, but another "lysozyme" didn't interest them. That this substance seemed to be destroying disease germs, not harmless ones, made little difference to them.

Fleming had already shown, however, that he could carry on without encouragement. So he began to investigate his new find on his own. He had the mold plate photographed for future reference. Then he took a bit of the mold and transferred it to a tube of fresh broth. Over the next several days the mold grew, forming a thick mat on the surface. The solution beneath the mold turned bright yellow. Fleming mixed some of this "mold juice" with melted agar. He cut a shallow gutter across the surface of a sterile agar plate and filled the ditch with the yellow mixture. Now he streaked different kinds of bacteria across the trough and incubated the culture.

The results of the experiment must have pleased Fleming. For while a few types of disease germs were unaffected and grew abundantly in thick streaks right up to the gutter of mold juice, a number of other kinds were destroyed; they disappeared near the trough. The juice had some power to kill them. It seemed to be a strange, new antiseptic that worked against certain harmful germs, germs that

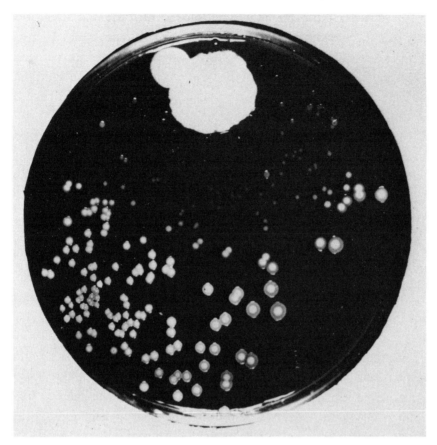

Fleming's original culture plate of Penicillium. *Note how few and faint are the colonies of bacteria in the area around the patch of mold at the top center of the petri dish. Typical colonies of germs are seen a distance away in the lower half of the plate.*

caused pneumonia, scarlet fever, meningitis, diphtheria, and gonor-rhea.

More than fifty years earlier, Pasteur had suggested that the day might come when harmless microorganisms might be used to destroy harmful ones. And, in 1889, another Frenchman, P. Vuillemin, had given this possibility the name "antibiosis." But the first attempt to put this idea to practical use as a treatment for people had failed. And critics of antibiosis argued convincingly that any natural agent powerful enough to destroy other life would likely harm the body as well. This was the same logic that had been used against chemotherapy before Salvarsan.

Now Fleming had come upon this mold that could kill disease germs. What an excellent antiseptic it might make. But would this example of antibiosis prove to be poisonous to people? Fleming knew that it was one thing for the mold's juice to dissolve germs on a culture plate and quite another for it to do so safely in an infected wound. He was encouraged, however, to learn more about this peculiar mold. It proved to be a strain of penicillia, a common enough group of molds found on ripening cheese, stale bread, and rotting fruit. The mold's name comes from the Latin word *penicillus,* which means "brush." Under a microscope, the mold looks like a tiny dust brush. So Fleming called the powerful mold juice "penicillin."

Fleming made a number of cultures of the mold and continued to experiment with its bright yellow juice. He found that penicillin killed germs even when greatly diluted. It killed them when mixed with human blood without destroying the white blood cells. Here, then, was a powerful natural agent much safer than the chemical antiseptics. To prove it was not poisonous in other ways, Fleming injected penicillin into a healthy rabbit and a mouse, and there were no ill effects. He also used it safely to clear up an eye infection in one of the laboratory assistants.

But what kind of substance was penicillin? Could it be purified? Fleming needed the help of chemists to extract pure penicillin from the mold juice. Only then could a measured amount, a dose, be relied upon to produce an effect. But Almroth Wright had no chemists on his staff. So Fleming asked two students in his department, Stuart Craddock and Frederick Ridley, to try to purify penicillin. In the

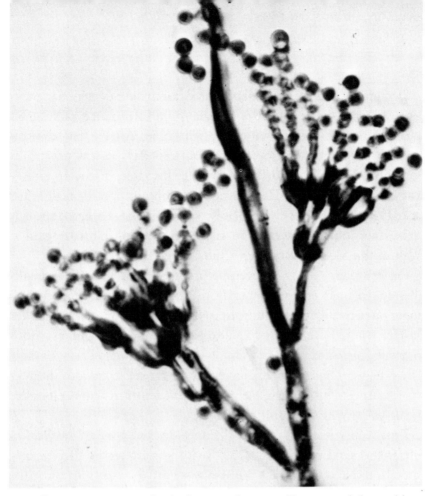

Penicillium notatum. *Under high magnification, filaments of the mold resemble small dust brushes.*

overcrowded wing, the two students were forced to work at a sink in a drafty hallway.

Craddock and Ridley found that the yellow color of the mold juice was due to an impurity. But try as they did for many months, they could not separate pure penicillin from other substances in the extract. Finally, they were left with a brown, sticky mess that looked like "melted toffee" (candy). Frustrated and discouraged, the earnest young men decided against publishing their efforts—an unfortunate decision, as it turned out.

Fleming, of course, was disappointed not to have penicillin in purer form. It took about five days for the mold to produce its valuable juice—and then the substance was unstable. After a few days its strength began to fade; by ten to fourteen days it was practically powerless. Fleming decided to announce his latest discovery, but he was on shaky ground. He had failed to obtain pure penicillin and lacked knowledge of its exact chemistry. He must have believed strongly in its importance, however, to risk embarrassing himself again in front of the Medical Research Club.

On February 13, 1929, even before Craddock and Ridley finally abandoned their efforts to purify the extract, Fleming presented a paper on penicillin to the authoritative research body. The outspoken Pasteur would have aroused and excited this audience with his showmanship, but Alexander Fleming had none of Louis Pasteur's flair. The bright promise of penicillin faded in his self-conscious, humble speech. And to his misery, Fleming's audience once again responded to his paper with an insulting silence.

True to his reserved nature, Fleming showed none of the hurt he felt at this cold reception. (Only years later, after he had become famous, did he speak of it.) But, twice rebuffed by the scientific club, his enthusiasm for penicillin suffered. And it was frustrating to work with such an unstable substance. An agent so unreliable seemed far from the safe, practical antiseptic for which he had hoped.

Had Fleming only tested penicillin in sick animals instead of healthy ones, things might have turned out differently. He might have discovered that penicillin was far more important as a medicine to be taken internally to fight germ-caused diseases than merely as an antiseptic for surface infections. But Almroth Wright frowned upon experimenting with infectious germs in animals. Wright held that such experiments had little relationship to the treatment of sick humans, and Fleming respected his chief's views. He also shared Wright's basic conviction that cures for infectious diseases would come from progress in immunology—from vaccines, not from chemicals, even natural ones. So Fleming, who at first had been so excited by penicillin, began other work. He continued to grow the mold, but he used penicillin only as a tool to eliminate unwanted germs that contaminated his bacterial cultures. Research on penicillin came to a halt at St. Mary's.

In 1929, Fleming published the paper he had read to the indifferent Medical Research Club. Then he gathered together his notes on penicillin and placed them in his file. Though he made no further efforts to investigate penicillin, he obeyed the sacred rules of science: to keep clear, informative notes and to report one's findings. Thus, although the discoverer of penicillin did not realize the importance of what he had found and put it aside, he did light the torch that made it possible for others who might come along to find and develop the mold drug.

A biochemist named Harold Raistrick, an outstanding authority on the chemicals produced by molds, was told about penicillin by a colleague who had read Fleming's paper. Raistrick obtained a culture of the penicillin mold from Fleming and began to study it. He sent a bit of the fungus to an American expert, Charles Thom, for help in identifying it more precisely. The American reported that the mold was an exceedingly rare strain of *Penicillium*. He identified this particular strain as *Penicillium notatum*.

But although Raistrick had read Fleming's paper by now, he did not know that attempts already had been made to purify penicillin. Craddock and Ridley had never published their methods or their unsuccessful results. So, in 1931, Raistrick and his assistants unknowingly repeated Craddock and Ridley's work—with the same frustrating outcome. The stumbling block was penicillin's instability: the agent broke down, or changed, before it could be extracted. Though penicillin also defied Raistrick's efforts to obtain it in pure form, he did describe the problem and publish his work to guide others.

While Raistrick was struggling with the mold juice, a former student of Fleming's at St. Mary's wrote to him also to obtain a culture of *Penicillium*. Doctor C. G. Paine was studying disease germs at the University of Sheffield in England's great northern steel center. He too had read Fleming's paper and wished to investigate penicillin. Fleming, pleased by Paine's interest, gladly sent him a culture.

The younger bacteriologist had difficulty growing the mold, and the penicillin he obtained varied in strength. He tried to treat three hospital patients suffering from staphylococcal infections of the skin with it. But these trials were unsuccessful. He, nevertheless, tried penicillin again. Paine put the mold juice into the infected eyes of four babies. Two had gonorrheal infections, and two, staphylococcal. Three of the children were cured. He bathed a coal miner's infected eye with penicillin, and the infection cleared, permitting a surgeon to operate and remove a stone chip that threatened the man's vision.

Although Fleming had used mold juice to clear the eye infection of a laboratory assistant earlier, Paine was the first to give penicillin clinical trials. But he too failed to recognize its tremendous potential. Like Fleming, Paine thought of penicillin only as a surface antiseptic—one that was a bother to produce and too unstable to keep. It seemed impractical, an agent of too little value, to report on in scientific journals. So Paine did not publish his results.

Paine's interest in penicillin faded, and he went on to other work. He, like Fleming, had been at the brink of a major discovery without realizing it. Before he abandoned penicillin, however, Paine shared his experiments with the Chief of the Department of Pathology, that branch of medicine that studies the effects of diseases on people. The Pathology Department at Sheffield was headed at that time by a young Australian named Howard Walter Florey.

5

THE BUSHRANGER
TAKES CHARGE

In 1932, Howard Florey could not have imagined that he was to become one of the heroes of the penicillin story. When he first learned about the yellow mold juice from his colleague Dr. Paine, he was, in fact, equally unimpressed with the prospects for this unstable extract. Besides, chemotherapy had fallen back into disfavor among physicians. Doctors still regarded chemical agents that killed germs and fought infections with suspicion. So it is easy, then, to understand why Florey didn't bother to look into the mold juice. He missed out on an early opportunity to present the world with its first "wonder drug": penicillin. But Florey was to have a second chance—later.

Howard Florey had come to England from Australia on a Rhodes Scholarship, a prize awarded students outstanding in athletics as well as academic studies. He had entered Oxford University in 1922 to pursue a career in medical research. (At that time, Alexander Fleming was working on lysozyme at St. Mary's.)

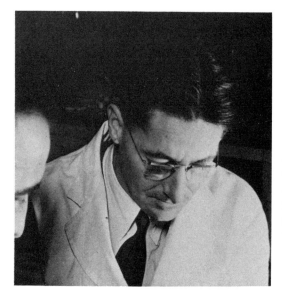

Howard Florey, when he came to England from Australia in 1922, could not have imagined that he was to become a hero in the penicillin story.

Florey did excellent work at Oxford and began to attract the attention of important scientists. One of these was Sir Charles Sherrington, who contributed greatly to the knowledge of how the body functions. Sherrington selected the young Australian to become an assistant, a great honor. But Florey had a way of minimizing his own achievements. In a typical comment to his girlfriend, Ethel Hayter Reed, a medical student back in Australia, he wrote that he felt like a "dud" in research but would try doing it for a year.

Florey did that year—and then another. He worked hard for Sherrington, who became fond of Florey and took special interest in him. Sherrington guided Florey into the field of Pathology and sent him on to Cambridge, Britain's other great old university. Florey remained at Cambridge for a year and then was given an opportunity to go to the United States on a Rockefeller Foundation Fellowship to do medical research in New York City. Florey accepted. As it developed, however, Florey spent most of his time studying under Professor Alfred Newton Richards at the University of Pennsylvania in Philadelphia. Richards was one of America's great pharmacologists, an expert on medications. Florey's earnest efforts made an impression on Richards that would, in the future, affect the development of penicillin.

The following year, 1926, back in England, Florey was joined by his Australian sweetheart, Ethel, and they married. Florey and Ethel moved on first to Cambridge, and then to Sheffield. It was at Sheffield that he learned about penicillin from Paine. Florey rose rapidly through the academic ranks. When a vacancy occurred in the prestigious post of Chief of the Sir William Dunn School of Pathology at Oxford, Florey applied for it.

Excellently qualified people were competing for the prized position at Oxford. Finally, the selection board had narrowed down the choice of candidates to Florey and another, more conservative, scientist. The board deliberated and just about decided to appoint the other man

The Sir William Dunn School of Pathology where the Oxford team developed penicillin

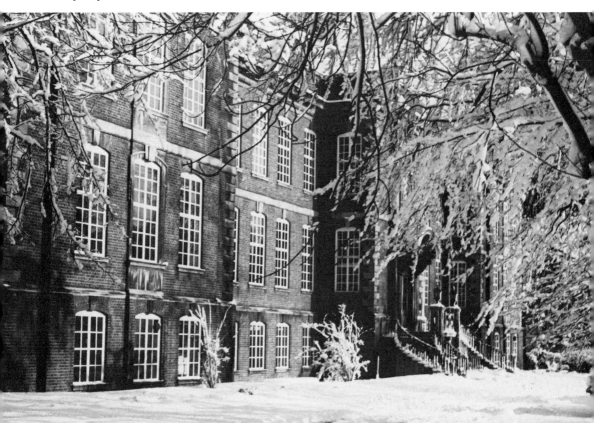

when their meeting was interrupted by the late arrival of an important member. This powerful and influential person was Sir Edward Mellanby, Secretary of the esteemed Medical Research Council. Fortunately for Florey, both he and Mellanby had been at Sheffield together, and Mellanby respected Florey's drive and ability. Mellanby was convinced that Florey could modernize the pathology department, and he persuaded the board to appoint Florey.

In only thirteen years, the energetic, ambitious young Australian had risen to one of the top positions in medical science, a remarkable achievement for a man only thirty-seven years old. And while Florey, his wife, their young daughter, and infant son were settling into life at Oxford, important changes were taking place in Europe.

It was now 1935. Benito Mussolini, the Italian dictator, defied the League of Nations, the international organization formed to keep the peace after World War I. Italian troops invaded Ethiopia in East Africa. In Germany, Adolph Hitler and the Nazi Party, having already risen to power, were busily building powerful military forces. The Nazis also had started a campaign of persecution against Jews, many of whom left Germany. Among these refugees were several gifted scientists.

At Elberfeld, in Germany, a physician-scientist named Gerhard Domagk was following in the footsteps of Paul Ehrlich. Domagk, too, searched among the dyes for chemicals that would destroy germs. Like Ehrlich before him, he screened compound after compound for antibacterial activity and methodically tested one after another on laboratory animals. It was tedious work. Almroth Wright visited Domagk's laboratory at one point and left convinced that such "groping in the dark" was wasteful and foolish.

But Domagk's efforts paid off. Among the chemicals he tested, he found a bright red dye that was effective against streptococci, germs that cause scarlet fever and other serious diseases. The chemical cured laboratory mice infected with these harmful germs. Domagk called his discovery Prontosil.

While Domagk was working with Prontosil, his daughter one day happened to puncture her finger with a knitting needle. The wound became infected with streptococci. The usual methods of care failed to help, and the infection spread. The girl's condition became desperate. Domagk considered using Prontosil. But the drug had never been tested on people, and he had no way of knowing if it was safe. His daughter was dying, however, so, as a last resort, he gave her the drug. To his joy and relief, the infection cleared and the girl recovered.

News of Prontosil spread rapidly. Within the year, two French chemists at the Pasteur Institute in Paris identified the active agent in Prontosil as a chemical belonging to a group called the sulfonamides. Chemical companies quickly realized how profitable sulfonamides might become and began a race to develop them. They produced new forms of these sulfa drugs to patent and sell. A patent set down the formula of a drug and registered it in the name of the pharmaceutical company that made it. The patent gave the company an exclusive right to make and sell that medicine.

As the new sulfa drugs became more available and were tested more widely, they proved to be effective against streptococcal infections, from sore throats to deadly childbed fever. They also fought the germs that caused meningitis and other bacterial diseases.

The sulfa drugs did not kill germs on contact like antiseptics but instead interfered with the germs' growth and development. The drugs could be used in a variety of ways: as a powder sprinkled into wounds, or as a liquid to be injected, or as a pill to be taken by mouth. The sulfa drugs proved once and for all the value of chemical agents in fighting infections both on the surface and inside the body. They were a major breakthrough. Though there remained a host of disease germs that were unaffected by sulfa drugs, these laboratory-made medicines renewed interest in chemotherapy.

The first wave of excitement about the sulfa drugs was a powerful stimulus to medical scientists everywhere. It stirred Howard Florey.

But the recently appointed Chief of the Sir William Dunn School of Pathology at Oxford found that he had inherited a dying department. The newly constructed, splendidly equipped red-brick building was like a tomb that stood empty and unused. Money problems plagued the department; it was severely understaffed, and its few laboratory technicians, lacking direction, often gathered in a basement room around a barrel of beer.

Florey was determined to improve the department. He worked diligently from the moment he arrived each day, and could be seen at his laboratory bench, steel-rimmed glasses perched on his long, lean face, working with such concentration that he inspired everyone. Florey had an amazing capacity to carry on five or six different lines of research at one time. And his energy and spirit were contagious. He was also respected for his honesty and fair-mindedness. The department's morale improved, and the beer barrel disappeared. Now there was always work to be done.

Florey was creating an outstanding research center with his enthusiasm for work and his ideas. He enjoyed experimentation most of all. He was fond of saying that if you did an experiment you might not always find an answer, but if you did not experiment, you could be certain not to find one. Florey also realized that biomedical research had advanced to a point beyond the skills of any one scientist. So he set out to bring together experts in bacteriology, biochemistry, and pathology to work as a research team.

Penicillin, by this time, had faded from Florey's thoughts. But such was fate that he was fascinated with Fleming's other discovery, lysozyme, the curious substance that dissolves harmless bacteria. Florey had been studying its properties for years. Now he had come to the barrier that had frustrated Fleming. He could not purify lysozyme; he needed a biochemist.

One of the first people Florey recruited, therefore, was 29-year-old Ernst Boris Chain, a biochemist. Chain was a German-Jewish

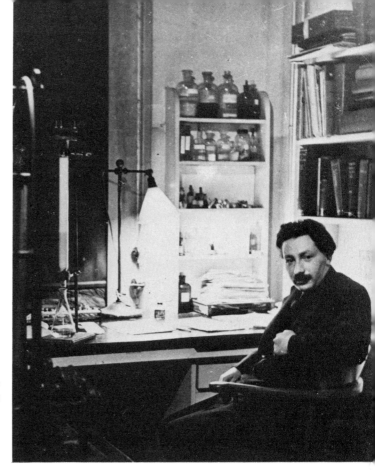

Dr. Ernst Chain in his laboratory at Oxford, about 1940

refugee from Berlin who had left Germany in 1933, on the day Adolph Hitler had risen to power. Chain had come to London, and thence to Cambridge. There he distinguished himself as a gifted worker. Chain was a short man with a dark mustache, friendly, and with much charm. He was also excitable and had the temperament more of someone in the arts than the usual scientist. In fact, he was an accomplished pianist.

No one could have predicted that two men, ten years apart in age and so different in personality as Ernst Chain and Howard Florey, would become good friends as well as successful collaborators. Unlike the younger, outgoing Chain, who enjoyed talking to people and made friends easily, Florey was reserved and difficult to know. When

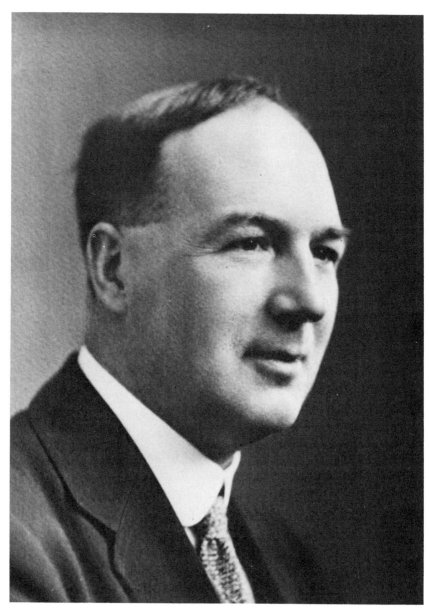

Sir Edward Mellanby, Secretary of the British Medical Research Council, whose powerful influence affected the development of penicillin

Florey spoke, he was blunt and had little grace. He had no ability at small talk or friendly conversation; he had trouble making friends. Yet Florey and Chain liked one another, and the two would take long walks together through the University Parks. The link between them may have been their shared ambition for scientific achievement.

In his first two years at Oxford, Chain completed a project he had begun at Cambridge on snake poisons and then went on to cancer research. But he needed help in isolating the minute amounts of substances he was studying. So he urged Florey to hire Dr. Norman G. Heatley, whom he had known at Cambridge. Heatley was an ingenious laboratory engineer skilled in micro-methods, the techniques for separating tiny cell structures and substances. He was a wizard at inventing instruments and equipment for his work. With the help of Edward Mellanby and the Medical Research Council, funds were granted in 1936 for Heatley's appointment.

Money problems, however, continued to hamper Florey's efforts to improve the department. Britain was in an economic depression and funds for research were scarce. The Medical Research Council had to ration its grants carefully. The pathology department at Oxford was put on a strict budget. Florey insisted that every penny possible be saved; he even cut down on heating and required that lights be turned off whenever possible. Still, Mellanby, representing the Research Council, often made unscheduled visits to the department to check on how its funds were being spent. This distraction irritated the department's busy scientists, many of whom resented Mellanby's intrusions and found him overbearing. Sometimes there were sharp exchanges between Mellanby and staff members.

Florey did his best to satisfy Mellanby. He recognized that it was important to please this influential man who had won him his appointment and now controlled the department's purse strings. Florey, no doubt, would have preferred to continue his research than to escort Mellanby about. Besides, diplomacy did not come easily to

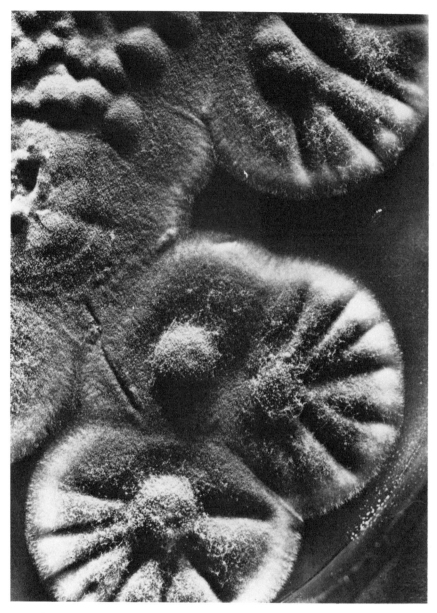

Penicillium notatum *growing on the surface of a petri-dish culture, magnified several times*

Florey. His proper, upper-class British colleagues, in fact, nicknamed Florey "the bushranger." This is an Australian term for an outlaw, or backwoodsman.

In 1937, the Oxford team, as it came to be known, succeeded in purifying lysozyme, and a year later Chain proved that it was an enzyme, as Fleming had suspected. Chain now became interested in antibiosis, in natural substances that exhibited antibacterial behavior. He collected some two hundred examples from the scientific literature. But Chain could find almost nothing describing the structure or chemical action of these substances. Then, early in 1938, he came across Fleming's paper on penicillin. The mold juice interested him.

Chain proposed to Florey that they undertake a research study on antibiotic substances, among them, penicillin. Florey agreed. By this time, the glowing promise of the antibacterial sulfa drugs had dimmed. The sulfas turned out to be ineffective in the presence of pus, and this limited their value. They also were found to have some harmful effects. These ranged from troublesome skin rashes to persistent vomiting to severe liver and kidney damage. So, with work on lysozyme winding down, Florey and Chain turned their attention to antibiosis.

By some extraordinary good luck there happened to be a culture of Fleming's mold on hand at the Dunn School. So Chain probably started his work on antibiosis with penicillin because the mold was already there and available. Chain discussed the project with Florey, and the two men agreed that penicillin, like lysozyme, would almost certainly turn out to be an enzyme, too. They decided that Chain would grow the mold and purify its juice, if he could. Then Florey would study penicillin's antibacterial action to learn how it worked. Florey and Chain's interest in penicillin at this point was probably academic, but the thought that they might develop a new medicine may have been in the back of their minds.

6

WAR COMES

IN the spring of 1938, the dark clouds of war were gathering over Europe. German troops marched into Austria. The peace that had followed World War I was coming apart. In Great Britain and elsewhere, people sensed that war was approaching. But Neville Chamberlain, the British Prime Minister, was determined to save the peace. So he went to Munich, Germany, in September to meet with Adolph Hitler and the Nazi leader's partner, Benito Mussolini. Could he reach an agreement with them? Chamberlain's goal was "peace in our time."

Hitler's price for peace was to acquire part of Czechoslovakia. England and France must stand aside and allow this further German expansion. Chamberlain submitted to Hitler's terms. He returned home to England convinced he had prevented war. But few people believed that Hitler and Mussolini would be content for long. Indeed, in March, 1939, Germany violated the agreement; her troops moved on to occupy all of Czechoslovakia. Then Italy, Germany's ally, invaded its tiny neighbor, Albania. The Munich Pact was worthless. Britain began to prepare for war.

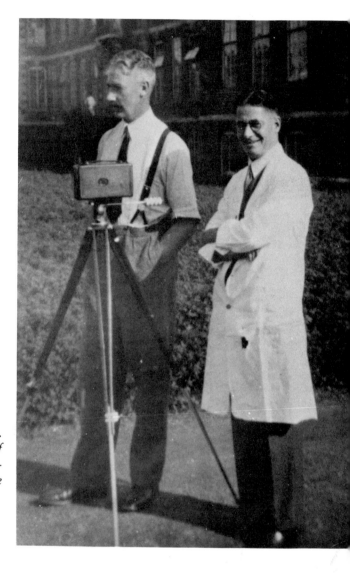

Howard Florey (right) and A. Q. Wells, a colleague, filming the staff as they dig air raid trenches behind the Dunn School early in the war, in 1939

The threat of war touched every corner of British life. A program for civil defense hurriedly began. If war came, German bombs would likely fall on Britain. So the government issued gas masks to every citizen and ordered that air-raid shelters be dug, first-aid stations prepared, and, finally, that air-raid drills, with wailing sirens, become routine practice. The whole population was put on alert.

At the Dunn School, the staff took turns from their regular research work to dig an air-raid shelter behind the red-brick building. Charles Florey, age four, the younger of the two Florey children, enjoyed watching the physicians and scholars swing picks and shovels like laborers.

Howard Florey, as head of his department, was responsible for certain emergency plans. He set up a blood bank for the Oxford area and was given use of a van for this purpose. His wife, Ethel, participated also. She took charge of organizing teams of physicians to obtain blood from donors. Though partially deaf, Dr. Ethel Florey, every bit as strong willed as her husband, did not allow her handicap to interfere with this work. She was pleased to have a role in the effort. Younger physicians in the program quickly learned to respect Ethel Florey for her tough, efficient, no-nonsense attitude toward work.

Meanwhile, Chain was having difficulty getting started with pen-

Howard Florey, his wife Ethel, and their two children, Paquita and Charles, about 1940

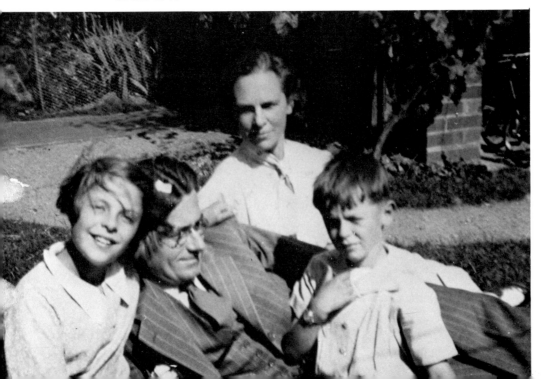

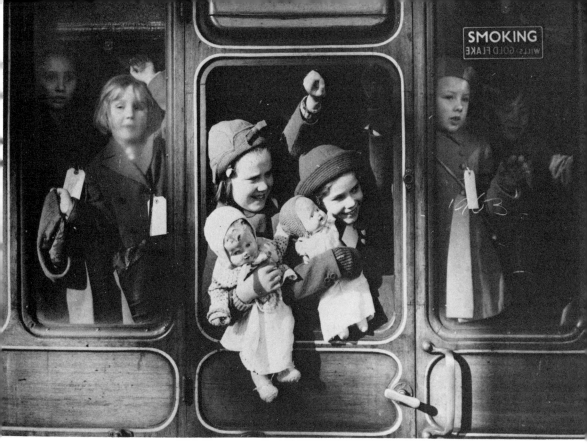

London children being evacuated from the city for safety in the British countryside

icillin. There were problems growing the mold. He relied heavily on the work Raistrick had published in 1932. But using Raistrick's method of growing the mold on synthetic broth in shallow petri dishes was very slow. It took months of patient effort to produce the first few droplets of penicillin.

In August, 1939, Britain began drafting young men into military service, and thousands flocked to enlist voluntarily. By August 31, war seemed so near that an extraordinary measure was announced. School children in London were to be separated from their parents and sent out to families in the countryside to safety. Bombing was expected. The evacuation took place on September 1, the next day.

London children reported to school with small suitcases, each containing a gas mask, a change of clothes, and a packet of food.

That day, September 1, 1939, Germany invaded Poland. The British and French insisted that Germany withdraw. Britain and France were committed by a treaty to defend Poland. But Germany ignored the British demand. So, on September 3, Britain and France declared war on Germany. The war that everyone feared began.

Britain committed her resources to the war effort. She sent troops to France, and, on the home front, sacrifice became the order of the day. Money was needed for the tools of war: guns, ships, planes, and tanks. Medical research was cut back and forced to get by on less. Florey's department at Oxford was already scrimping, and the prospect of further cuts worried the research-minded Australian. He realized that his continual haggling for funds was beginning to irritate Mellanby. But the new project on antibacterial substances that he and Chain were beginning seemed all the more important now because of the war.

So Florey risked appealing to Mellanby once more. This time he asked only for a modest hundred pounds, less than three hundred dollars, to continue their work. He promoted the new project enthusiastically. Florey predicted that penicillin could be produced easily in large amounts and purified without difficulty. He also proposed animal tests of penicillin and hinted for the first time of its possible value as a medicine.

It was most unusual for Florey, who was normally quite cautious, to anticipate such results, especially when research had barely begun. So it is likely that Chain's confidence and optimism influenced him. Whatever the case, Florey's letter to Mellanby on September 6, 1939, contained the first clue that he and Chain had begun to see that their work on penicillin might lead to a practical, antibacterial drug.

Mellanby's response was positive, but he offered Florey only twenty-five pounds, less than a hundred dollars, and, perhaps, one hundred

62

pounds more some time in the future. This was barely enough to proceed, and Florey was disappointed. With no other likely prospects for funding in England, the work on penicillin would stop. But Florey was never one to quit. So he turned now to the Rockefeller Foundation in New York City, the reknowned organization that had awarded him a fellowship fourteen years earlier. In fact, the Foundation had already given him support for his work on lysozyme. And so, with Chain's help, he drafted a broad research proposal that included the project on penicillin. He asked for five thousand dollars a year for at least three years to cover staff salaries and expenses, and roughly three thousand altogether for equipment.

Florey sent his letter to New York in November. The year, 1939, was drawing to an end. Britain, by now, was beginning to experience shortages brought on by the war. Food, clothing, and gasoline had become scarce and were rationed; every loyal citizen was learning to do with less and to accept this sacrifice as his duty. Florey, however, was unwilling to sacrifice his research; nor did he feel unpatriotic in seeking help in America. After all, England was fighting, she felt, to defend the entire free world, and the Americans were still safe and prospering.

In asking for foreign aid, however, Florey risked antagonizing the proud Mellanby and the Medical Research Council. So Florey did not inform them of his request, not even when the Rockefeller Foundation awarded him the funds needed and generously extended the term of the grant from three to five years. Now, for the first time since coming to Oxford, Florey's money concerns lifted; he could concentrate on research.

The war changed everyone's plans. One of those affected was Dr. Norman Heatley, the gifted young scientist from Cambridge, whom Florey had taken on to assist Chain. Heatley had won a Rockefeller Foundation fellowship to do research in Denmark. But because of the danger that all of Europe might become involved in the war,

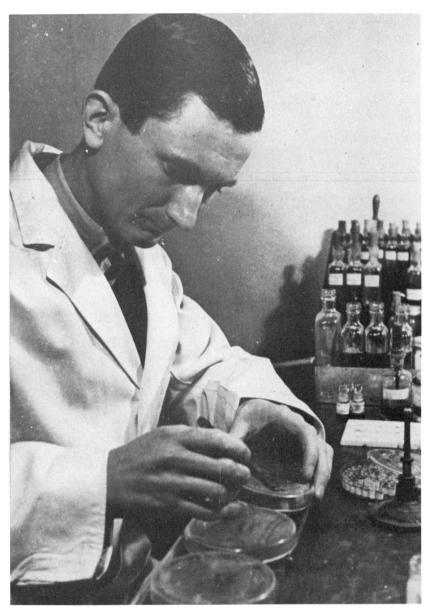

*Dr. Norman G. Heatley, the "wizard" of the penicillin team at Oxford, ·
marking petri-dish cultures*

Florey persuaded him to stay on at Oxford as his assistant.

Heatley's genius at improvising apparatus to solve laboratory problems quickly established him as an essential member of the Oxford team. He worked with Chain to improve the method for growing the mold and harvesting penicillin. Raistrick's technique required ten to twenty days. During that time, the mold in the petri dish formed a mat on the surface of the broth; the mold gradually changed color from white to blue-green. As it darkened, the pale broth beneath the fungus became yellow with penicillin.

Chain and Heatley experimented with the broth, adding substances to see if they could improve the mold's yield. Nothing seemed to work, but they learned that they could shorten the time it took the mold to produce penicillin by adding an extract of brewer's yeast. They also found that, by removing the broth when it had become bright yellow and replacing it with fresh broth, the mold would continue producing penicillin. This trick could be performed as many as twelve times. And they learned also that the mold did best when grown on broth of a particular depth. With this information, they turned from the shallow little petri-dish cultures to growing the mold in bottles laid on their sides. As a result, they produced more mold juice.

Heatley took charge of growing the mold, freeing Chain for other work on penicillin. And Chain discovered that penicillin was not an enzyme, like lysozyme, after all. Penicillin needed to be purified, however, before more could be learned about its chemical structure and action.

The same problems that had discouraged Raistrick when he attempted to extract penicillin from the mold juice now confronted Chain. Penicillin was unstable; it kept disappearing from the mold juice while Chain worked on it. Heatley came to his aid and achieved the first breakthrough at Oxford. Heatley used the chemical ether to extract penicillin from the mold juice. Then he used water to remove the penicillin from the ether. This was an important advance beyond Raistrick's method. But to keep the penicillin extract stable, it had to be kept cool. So Heatley set up a system of glass tubing and coils wrapped in crushed ice through which the solution could safely pass.

In March, 1940, using Heatley's system, the Oxford team finally obtained what they thought to be pure penicillin. They freeze-dried the extract to preserve it. Thousands of man hours and gallons of precious mold juice had finally yielded a tiny amount of dry, brown powder—hardly enough to cover the surface of a dime.

Now the hard-earned powder had to be tested. Would it be active against germs or had it lost its power during the extraction process? Carefully Chain dissolved a bit of the valuable powder in water and tested it on cultures of streptococci. To his delight, it proved to be much more powerful than the crude mold juice, more powerful also than the newest sulfa drugs, against the same germs. But would the purified penicillin be too strong to be used safely in animals?

Animal tests were Howard Florey's responsibility. But either Florey was too busy at the moment to conduct this test (as Chain later claimed) or Chain's eagerness for answers prompted him to go ahead on his own. He had two mice injected with the penicillin extract. Though this solution was infinitely stronger than the mold juice Fleming had tested years earlier, the mice came through the experiment healthy and unharmed. The test was one of the high points of the entire project for Chain, but it may have damaged his friendship with Florey. In his haste for answers, he had, perhaps, overstepped his bounds and offended his partner.

If Florey was put off when Chain told him of his success, however, it is likely that he did not openly express his feelings; that was not his nature. Instead, Florey took over what was left of the precious powder and, in his own careful, methodical way, repeated Chain's experiment to satisfy himself. The results were just as favorable. Florey went on to test penicillin in other mice and rats, rabbits and cats. In each case, penicillin proved safe. He learned too that the drug was excreted unchanged in the animal's urine. Florey also added penicillin to human blood and found that it did not harm white blood cells as antiseptics had.

Meanwhile, bacteriologists on the Oxford team tested the extract against a host of different disease-causing bacteria, checking Fleming's original work. They too found it effective against the germs that caused pneumonia, scarlet fever, meningitis, diphtheria, and gonorrhea. And, unlike the sulfa drugs, the presence of pus did not interfere with penicillin's action. Penicillin made germs swell and become misshapen. It prevented them from dividing and multiplying, and eventually caused them to burst and die.

The results of these tests excited the Oxford team. Could they possibly have in their hands an agent so powerful and safe that it could save millions of lives? The researchers turned to their work with a new sense of urgency. They knew, however, that the destruction by penicillin of disease germs in a petri dish did not necessarily ensure that penicillin would kill germs in living, sick animals. This was the critical experiment that Fleming, earlier, had not performed. Florey realized that this crucial test would determine the future of penicillin. He planned it for May 25, 1940.

7

THE FUNGUS FACTORY

WHILE the small group of scientists at Oxford were wondering if they might be on the brink of a major discovery, the war with Germany took a sudden, disasterous turn. German troops occupied Denmark; Norway fell. And on May 10, 1940, Nazi armored forces swept around the main French defenses and broke through into the heart of France. One column of German tanks and troops headed south toward Paris; another raced westward toward the English Channel to trap the British army in France. Meanwhile, Holland, Belgium, and Luxemburg were crushed. The war had become a nightmare.

These defeats forced the British Prime Minister, Neville Chamberlain, to resign. Winston Churchill, a short, tough plug of a man with a powerful and eloquent voice, took his place. The situation was grim. On a strip of beach in northwestern France, at Dunkirk, the beaten British and French armies gathered. The English Channel was at their backs, and they were trapped.

On Saturday, May 25, James Kent arose and dressed for work. It was a beautiful, sunny morning; a hint of

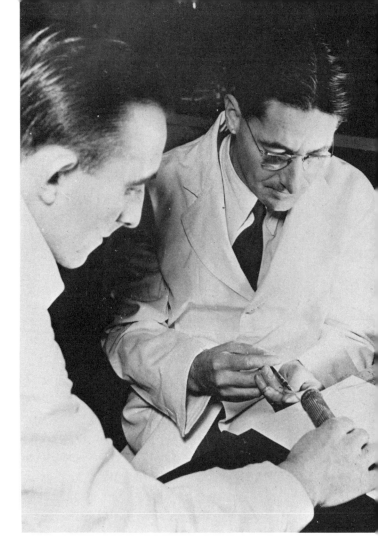

Florey injecting penicillin into the tail of a mouse confined temporarily in a tubular cage held by his loyal assistant, Jim Kent

early summer was in the air. It was odd to work at the laboratory on a Saturday, but Kent never thought of complaining. The war had changed many things; besides, he had worked for Howard Florey thirteen years now, ever since the professor took him on as his animal assistant back at Sheffield when Jim was only fourteen. When Florey moved to Oxford, he'd taken Jim along. No assistant was more loyal to his chief than Jim.

Kent went to the animal house adjoining the red-brick building at the Dunn School. Here were kept the animals needed for tests. He checked the mice that would be required in the experiment scheduled for that morning. Jim chose eight lively white ones, transferred them to special, glass-topped cages, and carried them over to Room 46, Dr. Florey's laboratory. There one of the bacteriologists was carefully setting out eight doses of deadly streptococci.

Florey arrived at 11:00 A.M. and began the experiment. While Jim held each of the eight mice, Florey injected them with the germs. Jim put four infected mice back in their cages. These would receive no penicillin; they would serve as standards, or controls, by which to judge the effect of penicillin. Florey divided the remaining four infected mice into two groups, A and B. One hour later, he gave the two mice in group A a dose of penicillin and returned them to their cages. Then he gave group B half that dose, but group B would receive this amount four more times during the next ten hours.

Florey and Kent observed the mice all afternoon. Nothing happened. Florey finally sent Jim home at 6:30 P.M.; then Heatley joined Florey to take up the watch. The untreated controls were beginning to look ill by now, but the treated mice seemed well. Florey gave the mice in group B their third dose of penicillin at 7:00 P.M. and the two men left to have their dinners. Florey returned at 10:00 P.M. to give the B mice their last injection of penicillin. He jotted a note to Heatley, saying that the control mice looked quite ill and that, except for one mouse that was not very lively, the treated mice still seemed fine. Then Florey went home to sleep.

At 11:00 P.M., Heatley returned to resume the watch. A short time later, the first of the untreated mice died. Then, one by one, each of the remaining three controls also died. It was 3:30 A.M. by now, and only the mice that had received penicillin were still alive. Heatley rechecked groups A and B once more, wrote down his observations, and left on his bicycle for home.

Norman Heatley was ordinarily a quiet, unexcitable person, but that night, riding home in the blacked-out town at four in the morning, his mind was whirling with what he had just observed. Penicillin worked against deadly germs in living animals. In his distraction, Heatley failed to see an air-raid warden on patrol and crashed right into the poor fellow. There were some unkind words and quick apologies, but nothing could dim Heatley's happy mood.

The next morning, on Sunday, May 26, 1940, Florey, Chain, and Heatley met at the laboratory to examine the results of the experiment. The control mice lay dead where they had fallen in their cages. But all the treated mice were alive. Penicillin had protected them, and it was safe! The three scientists—the modest, quiet Heatley; the practical, down-to-earth Florey; and the quick-witted, excitable Chain— rejoiced together. Florey observed that both groups, A and B, had done equally well despite the differences in their treatment. He would have to learn more about the exact dose and way to use penicillin in future tests. But for now he was excited by the success of the experiment. He cheerily telephoned another member of the team to announce that the results were like a "miracle."

Across the English Channel at Dunkirk on that memorable Sunday, however, a different kind of miracle was taking place. It was impressively called "Operation Dynamo." But the only thing impressive about the comic flotilla that braved the choppy Channel that day was its courage. British sailors and civilians assembled a fleet of motor launches, yachts, fishing vessels, ferries, and excursion boats, as well as naval ships, to evacuate the encircled troops at Dunkirk. While Royal Air Force planes flew overhead to protect it, this courageous, rag-tag navy sailed back and forth to France through bombs and shells for nine days to rescue 335,000 British and French soldiers from the Germans.

The miracle at Dunkirk cheered the British people, but it did not disguise their desperate situation. German military power seemed

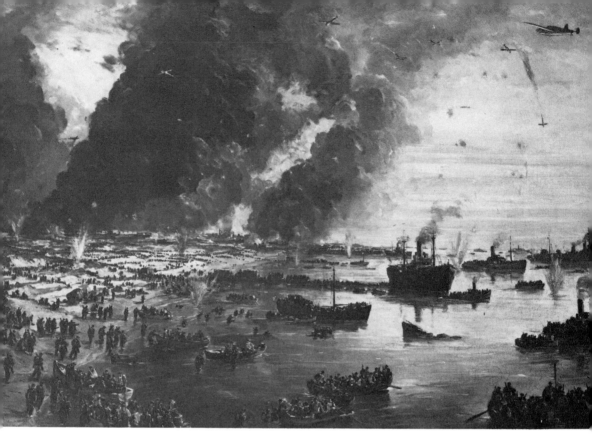

The miracle of Dunkirk. Remnants of the defeated British and French armies in France streaming onto British rescue vessels to escape capture by the Germans.

overwhelming. Britain stood alone now, and she had lost many troops and great quantities of arms and equipment in France. And Hitler was already suggesting that Britain surrender or face invasion. But the stirring voice of Winston Churchill inspired his people to fight on.

Britons went about their business with calm and courage. And Florey continued his work on penicillin. Fast on the heels of the first successful test, he began new experiments to learn more about how to use penicillin. These tests, however, required more penicillin than Heatley was able to produce in the bottles he was using. Penicillin was produced by fermentation, a process in which the mature mold gradually broke down into simpler substances, one of which was penicillin. But the yield was so small that much more mold needed to be grown to keep Florey supplied. So Heatley began growing the mold in every container he could get his hands on: pie plates, cookie tins, flasks, even a dog bath. He discovered that of all the unlikely containers he tried, penicillin grew quite happily in hospital bedpans.

Almost overnight the respectable Sir William Dunn School of Pathology at Oxford was turned into a hastily thrown-together production plant for penicillin. Every laboratory, office, nook, and cranny not needed for other projects became cluttered fermentation rooms for the blue-green fungus. And just then, when all this was happening, who should drop by but Sir Edward Mellanby on one of his unannounced visits to inspect the department! Whether Mellanby was on another of his ordinary snooping visits or had heard some rumor about unusual goings-on at the school, there was no hint. But there he was, curious as ever and totally in the dark about the all-out penicillin effort and the American monies that were funding it.

What a day poor Florey had. Pulled from his work, he had to escort Mellanby through the school and keep up a steady conversation to distract his guest. Florey guided the unsuspecting Mellanby down safe corridors and hurried him past hastily closed doors. And somehow, through all of this, he managed to divert Mellanby from the strange fumes that wafted through the building. He took Mellanby off to lunch as soon as he could. Then he had him escorted to his train. Had Mellanby learned of the extraordinary effort to produce penicillin at that point, the whole project might have been endangered. Because Mellanby was devoted to pure science, the sight of his dear pathology department being changed into a fungus factory might have enraged him.

For the next several weeks, Florey continued testing mice to find out more about the dosage and the effectiveness of penicillin. But still there was not enough extract to keep pace with the tests Florey needed to perform. So the shortage forced him to risk revealing his work. Florey went to a commercial laboratory and asked for help. But the firm he consulted was busy making vaccines and antitoxins to protect soldiers and civilians—and penicillin did not seem as important to the war effort. Florey was turned down.

On July 1, however, enough penicillin had been collected at Oxford to perform a mass experiment on fifty mice. With Jim Kent's help, Florey gave all the mice a large deadly dose of streptococci. Again, he left half the group untreated to serve as controls. Then, every three hours for the next two days and nights, he gave penicillin to the other twenty-five. The two men slept at the school, Kent on a cot in the laboratory and Florey in his study across the hall. An alarm clock woke them through the night to keep their schedule. After sixteen hours, the untreated mice were all dead. But twenty-four of the twenty-five mice that had received penicillin injections survived.

Florey tested penicillin next against other harmful germs, using mice. He tried it in mice infected with staphylococci. And, perhaps with the war in mind, he tested it against the deadly, wound-infecting, gas gangrene germs. Each time, penicillin proved to be effective in protecting infected mice.

Florey could see already that penicillin might be an extraordinary chemotherapeutic agent. For here was a substance of unequaled effectiveness against disease-causing germs—and it was not harmful to animal cells. This agent had a potential far beyond anything its discoverer, Fleming, had considered when he dismissed it as too impractical for use as a surface antiseptic. Here again was the same penicillin that Paine had mentioned to Florey at Sheffield eight years earlier. It was indeed as if fate had given Florey a second chance. He was determined to use it, this time. Florey planned to report the team's findings in *The Lancet*, Britain's medical journal.

While the team at Oxford assembled its notes for publication, German invasion barges gathered across the English Channel on the

French coast. German troops and tanks were massing to attack England. Britons prepared for the worst. Florey, Heatley, and others of the Oxford team were determined not to lose penicillin if the Germans came to Oxford. So, as a precaution, they rubbed the reproductive spores of the *Penicillium* mold into their clothes. These spores, like seeds, could remain dormant for a considerable time and then be activated to grow and reproduce the mold once more. Florey brushed the spores into the lining of his raincoat, producing a brown stain. Heatley rubbed them into the pockets of a suit. Somehow, if the invasion came, they hoped one of them might manage to escape and get to Canada or the United States to continue their work.

The likelihood that the villages and cities of Britain would soon become a battleground brought on other desperate measures. Many Britons sent their children away to safety in Canada and the United States. In July, 1940, 125 children of the faculty at Oxford left by ship for America. Among them were the Florey children, Paquita, age ten, and Charles, now five. They would spend the rest of the war with Dr. and Mrs. John Fulton in Connecticut. Fulton and Florey had been friends since their student days together at Oxford as Rhodes Scholars.

John Fulton traveled up to Montreal, Canada, to meet the Florey children. Through some mishap, they and other children had been dumped on the docks there in a confusion of baggage, officials, and newspaper reporters. But, like their parents, Paquita and Charles were unflappable and calm. Amidst the hubbub of people trying to sort matters out, there sat Paquita enjoying the comics, a pleasure she had never been permitted at Oxford.

During the summer of 1940, the German air force pounded British ports and airfields in preparation for the invasion. Then the Germans turned their attention to Britain's cities. London, Liverpool, and Manchester, but especially London, England's capital, were bombed. Waves of German bombers struck at Britain's industrial and popu-

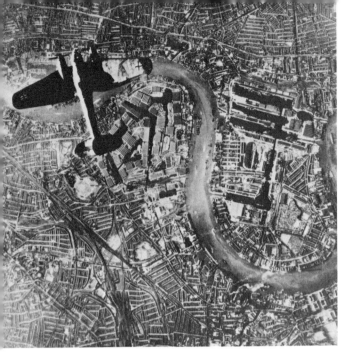

Battle of Britain. A German bomber aircraft over the Thames River, London.

Battle of Britain. Londoners take refuge in an underground railway station during an air raid, September 25, 1940.

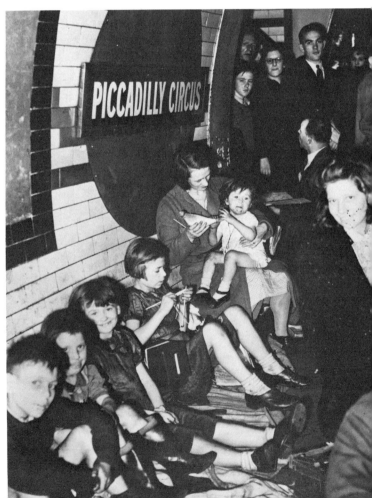

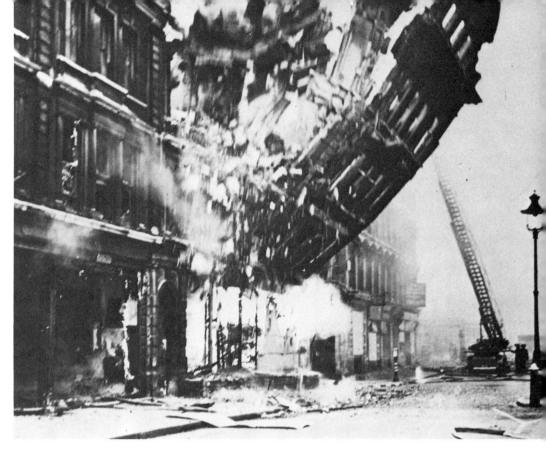

Battle of Britain. Bombs collapse a London building on May 11, 1941, during the blitz.

lation centers repeatedly. The Battle of Britain, as it came to be called, was fought in the air overhead and not on the beaches. Germany had three or four times the number of airplanes as the British. But the British had developed radar, which enabled them to detect enemy aircraft and to intercept them. The young pilots of the Royal Air Force fought with incredible courage to protect their island nation.

On August 24, 1940, while the blitz, the German air attacks, continued, a paper appeared in *The Lancet* entitled: "Penicillin As A Chemotherapeutic Agent." True to his sense of fairness, Florey listed the authors, seven members of the team including himself, not according to academic rank but by alphabetical order. The paper

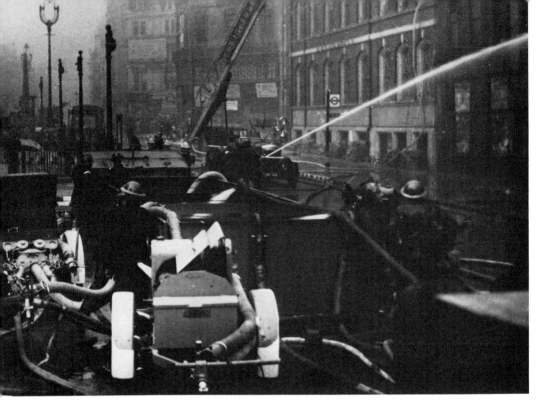

Battle of Britain. On a street in central London, firemen struggle to limit the damage after a bombing raid.

Battle of Britain. Civilian rescue workers, Britain's troops during the bombings, are shown removing an injured man who had been buried in debris for fourteen hours.

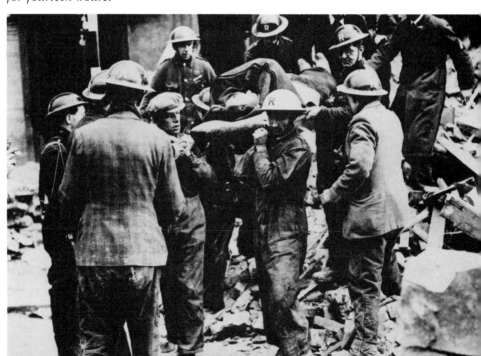

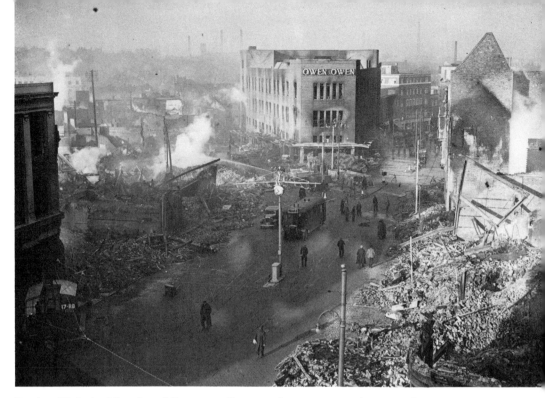

Battle of Britain. The city of Coventry digs out after an air attack, November 14, 1940.

reported that the group had found a way to purify and preserve penicillin. It went on to tell of penicillin's antibacterial effectiveness and safety in mice. The authors expressed gratitude to the American Rockefeller Foundation and to the British Medical Research Council for their support.

But if Florey had expected to arouse scientific interest in penicillin by publishing his findings, he must have been disappointed by how little reaction he stirred. Mellanby, of course, reacted quickly. And angrily. He accused Florey of giving too much credit to the Americans for their help. And when Florey reminded him of why the Oxford team had had to turn to the Rockefeller Foundation for aid, and how the project could not have continued without it, Mellanby was no happier.

Another unexpected result of *The Lancet* article was that Alexander Fleming telephoned to ask if he might come to Oxford to see what was being done. When Florey told Chain of the call, Chain was amazed. All along he had assumed that Fleming had died years earlier. On September 2, 1940, Alexander Fleming, now a white-haired, distinguished-looking man of fifty-nine, called at the Sir William Dunn School to inspect the project.

Florey greeted Fleming and introduced him to Chain. The Oxford scientists escorted Fleming on a tour of their facilities and explained the production process to him. But beyond some brief comment about "my old penicillin," Fleming said little. He finally left, taking with him a precious gift from Florey, a tiny sample of extract. But during his visit, Fleming had not uttered one word of praise or admiration for the team's achievements, nor had he congratulated them. Perhaps he was filled with remorse that he had not gone far enough with penicillin himself.

To Florey, the most disappointing result of the paper in *The Lancet* was the failure of any pharmaceutical company to show interest in penicillin. None of them contacted him to discuss producing it. So Florey followed up the publication by calling upon them. He learned that the British drug companies were already operating to their fullest capacities and were hard pressed to supply enough conventional medicines to the armed forces and to civilian hospitals and aid stations. Britain was under seige and suffering heavy casualties from the relentless bombings. The streets of London and other cities were the front lines of the war, and air-raid wardens, ambulance drivers, rescue workers, and firemen were the troops.

Florey realized that he could not persuade pharmaceutical companies to start large-scale, expensive production of an experimental drug at this time without impressive evidence first that it worked in humans. He had to proceed to testing penicillin on people. The problem, of course, was that production at Oxford barely provided enough extract for experiments on mice. Somehow, a way had to be found to increase the yield of penicillin. So Florey consulted Heatley, and the two of them designed a new container to grow the mold. Based on their success with growing the mold in bedpans, they came up with a rectangular vessel with a lid and side spout that could hold much more mold. Next, Florey searched for a factory that was not totally committed to war production. Finally he managed to get six hundred ceramic pots of the type he needed manufactured.

To get the pots delivered, however, presented another problem. Transportation in Britain was severely limited by gasoline rationing. All unessential travel was discouraged. So Norman Heatley found himself pressed into the role of truck driver, and he borrowed a lorry from Florey's civilian defense blood bank. Two days before Christmas, on December 23, 1940, mild, scholarly Heatley drove the truck a hundred miles to the factory to get the first 170 clay pots. He drove over rutted, icy, unfamiliar roads through snow, straining to find his way because all road signs had been removed in anticipation of German landings. Worst of all, Heatley had to ease along slowly on his return trip, lest a bump crack his valuable clay cargo. This harrowing, freezing, 200-mile round trip took almost eleven hours.

The push to produce penicillin for human testing was on, and there wasn't a moment to lose. Florey and others in the Oxford team were aware by this time that penicillin might make a great difference in treating the war wounded and save lives. So Florey, Heatley, and another member of the team spent Christmas eve and Christmas day getting the first vessels into production. They washed the pots, filled them with broth, sterilized them, and added the mold spores. Finally, they stacked the flat vessels into a heated room and began the incubation process. By the time Heatley had completed two more trips, delivered all the new containers, and put them into production, the Sir William Dunn School had literally become a full-time penicillin factory.

Heatley now tried to improve the extraction process. He tinkered

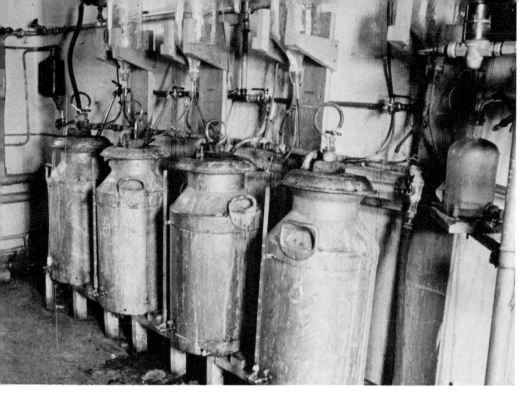

Heatley's wizardry. Part of the improvised apparatus to extract penicillin from the mold juice utilized milk cans.

and tested and finally concocted an incredible device. It consisted of yards of glass tubing, filters, sprays, pumps, a maze of plumbing, even signal lights and bells. His new contraption was so strange that it seemed more worthy of the Wizard of Oz than a serious scientist. But it handled the increased volume of mold juice better. It sped up the separation of penicillin from impurities after the mold juice was filtered. And it produced the most powerful penicillin yet. The delicate extract, however, had to be cooled as it was processed, so much of the procedure was carried out now in sub-zero temperatures in a cold room.

Florey hired six young women to assist with penicillin production. Because growing the mold spores required perfectly clean conditions, they wore rubber gloves and sterile white gowns, caps, and masks to prepare the pots. And because the floors were coated with oil to keep the dust down, they also wore galoshes. When the women worked in the cold extraction room, however, they were forced to wear thick, warm overcoats, gloves, woolen hats, and fur-lined boots. These women did their work cheerfully and diligently, and the efforts of these "Penicillin Girls," as they came to be known, added greatly to the production of the extract.

Within weeks, by the middle of January, 1941, Florey had enough penicillin on hand to set some aside for Chain to begin research on a synthetic way to produce penicillin. He also had enough to perform the next, all-important test—the first trial in a human being.

The Penicillin Girls carefully tending ceramic pot cultures of the mold at Oxford in 1941

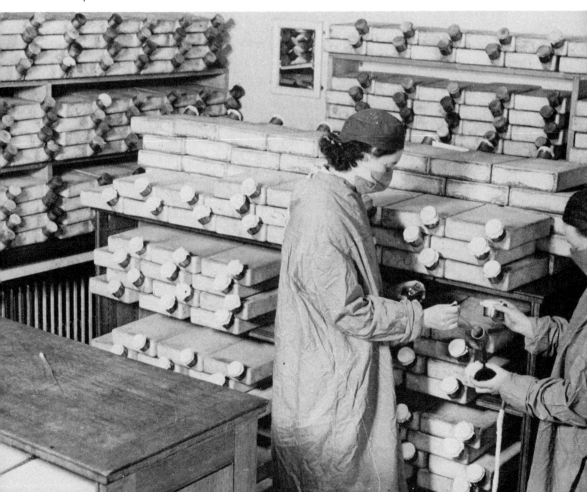

8

THE MIRACLE DRUG

THE great torchbearers of medical science—people like Jenner, Pasteur, Lister, Koch, Ehrlich, and all others who are responsible for progress—must sooner or later face the crucial test. They must try their discoveries on human beings. Florey had come to this turning point with penicillin. Now it was up to some ordinary person to take the risk that might make progress possible. Someone had to receive penicillin to prove that it was safe. This brave individual was Elva Akers.

Elva Akers, a woman in her forties from Oxford, knew she was dying. The cancer that had begun in her breast had spread throughout her body, and nothing could be done. When she was asked to volunteer for penicillin, she knew that the new drug she would be testing would not benefit her. But it might help doctors to perfect a cure for other diseases. So with nothing to gain but the satisfaction that she could help in the effort to save others, Mrs. Akers agreed to participate in the experiment.

The test took place on January 17, 1941. Within two hours after receiving the penicillin injection, Elva Akers developed chills and fever. This reaction worried Florey. The penicillin he was using must still have impurities. So Chain and another member of the team set to work to refine the extract further. They used a new method to purify the hard-earned brown powder. This yielded a yellow sediment, a purer penicillin. Other patients volunteered to try the purer drug; they suffered no ill effects. (This was a remarkable bit of luck, though no one realized it at the time. It later turned out that this newest extract still contained many impurities. It was only about 2.5 percent pure.)

Confident now that he had a safe extract to use, Florey felt ready to test the effectiveness of penicillin as an antibacterial medicine. He found a sick Oxford policeman to try it on. Albert Alexander, forty-three, had become ill as a result of a scratch at the side of his mouth from a rose thorn. The wound had become infected with staphylococci and then with streptococci—germs against which penicillin had worked so well experimentally in mice. The deadly bacteria had spread, forming pockets of pus on the policeman's scalp and in his eyes. Doctors drained these abscesses, but it did little good. They tried sulfa drugs, but these were ineffective in the presence of the pus. Alexander's condition steadily worsened. His left eye had to be removed. The infection spread to his bones, to his right shoulder, and then to his lungs.

Albert Alexander was near death on February 12, 1941, when he began receiving penicillin. The first dose was given by injection; then a solution of penicillin was dripped slowly into his veins. The precious drug, so short in supply, was rapidly excreted by the policeman's kidneys. His kidneys removed it so quickly that giving Alexander penicillin, Florey observed, was "like trying to fill a bath with the plug out."

So the dying policeman's urine was collected. It was saved in bottles and taken back to the laboratory by bicycle. There Chain, Heatley, or another member of the team extracted the drug for use again.

Ethel Florey and others took turns pedaling the urine back from the hospital to the laboratory. Local people, watching the scientists carrying the valuable urine through the streets of Oxford, nicknamed them the "P-patrol."

Penicillin had a dramatic effect on the policeman. In less than twenty-four hours, Alexander took a turn for the better. As the treatment continued, his fever disappeared, his abscesses improved, and his appetite returned. But after three days, the team's entire supply of penicillin was gone, and the only source for the drug was the ever-dwindling amount that could be saved from the policeman's urine. In two more days, even that was used up. Alexander continued to make some gains after the treatment ended, however, and the Oxford team hoped he could now fight off the infection on his own. But, in another week, Alexander was worse. The infection had flared up again. The team watched helplessly as the germs attacked the policeman's lungs once more. On March 15, a month after the start of the penicillin treatment, Albert Alexander died.

Alexander's death upset the scientists who had fought to save him. Their confidence in penicillin, however, was not diminished. They were certain that, had enough penicillin been available to continue treatment longer, they could have saved the policeman. And five days' use of the new extract had produced no harmful side effects. Still, the tragedy affected Florey's plans. He would not try penicillin on another person until he was sure he had enough to complete the treatment. And to be doubly certain, he would treat children, if possible, because a child, he reasoned, would need a smaller dose of the scarce extract than an adult.

The problem of getting enough penicillin to conduct adequate tests of the drug had ironies. The small, makeshift plant at Oxford could not produce the amount of extract that Florey needed. For this, commercial production was required. But no drug manufacturer would be willing to risk money to produce the drug for large-scale testing until there was sufficient evidence of its value. Somehow, Florey had to scrape together enough penicillin from his limited plant for a few more trials. The death of the Oxford policeman had overshadowed penicillin's worth in his case. What Florey needed were clear-cut successes to prove penicillin's value.

The next patient to be treated was a fifteen-year-old boy. The teenager had developed a streptococcal infection at the place where a pin had been inserted to fix a broken hip. The boy was seriously ill and running a high fever. The team gave him a small dose of penicillin every three hours. By the third day of treatment, the patient was greatly improved. But later, when the pin was removed, the infection reappeared. The dose of penicillin given had proven to be too small. Inexperience in judging how much penicillin to use had deprived Florey again of the cure he had hoped for.

An adult laborer with a large, painful boil on his back was the next person to receive penicillin. Such pus-filled infections usually required surgical treatment and took weeks to improve, leaving permanent scars. But penicillin cleared up the laborer's problem in a few days. Florey had a cure. But still, the case was not important enough to prove penicillin's worth. The laborer's boil could have been treated surgically.

The fourth case was heartbreaking. Four-and-a-half-year-old Johnny Cox had become desperately ill after measles spots on his left eyelid became infected. The infection spread through the eye socket and into the brain. Sulfa drugs failed, and Johnny lay in a coma, near death, when he started receiving penicillin. Within a few days on the drug, however, the child was remarkably better. Soon he was happily playing with toys and talking. And when penicillin was stopped, Johnny continued to improve. The case seemed to be just the kind of clear-cut proof Florey was seeking.

But then, suddenly, Johnny vomited; he lost consciousness and had a seizure. Penicillin was started again, but this time Johnny did not respond. In a few days, the child was dead. An autopsy, an examination after death, revealed that Johnny died from a hemorrhage into the brain; a blood vessel, weakened by the infection, had burst, killing him. The examination also showed, however, that the infection itself had been cleared up completely. The value of penicillin in this case was proven despite the unfortunate death of the patient.

Penicillin was used next to treat a 14½-year-old boy who was dangerously ill with a staphylococcal infection. The bacteria had entered his left hip joint and leg bone; it moved through his bloodstream to also attack his kidneys. Sulfa drugs and surgical treatment did not help. Penicillin was started and given for two weeks. The treatment was remarkably effective. The boy made an excellent recovery. And a similarly successful outcome was obtained in the sixth case, the treatment of a six-month-old baby with a severe urinary-tract infection. These last two patients amazed hospital attendants familiar with the usual outcomes in such serious cases. Penicillin was now openly spoken of as a "miracle" drug.

Florey and the members of his Oxford team collected their notes to publish another report in *The Lancet*. They wrote up their work, describing how they had produced and refined penicillin, their tests on animals, and the trials on six human beings. But Florey knew that these human trials were too few to establish the value of the drug. The proof he needed would require a great number of human tests. He had to obtain more penicillin.

Florey went once more to the pharmaceutical industry for help, and several drug companies responded by sending representatives up to Oxford to inspect the scientists' work. When they saw the complicated method that Heatley had devised to produce the mold drug, however, they lost interest. They realized that the fermentation-extraction process would be very costly to start up and manage, and that, in the meantime, a cheaper chemical means of producing the drug synthetically might come along to compete with them. Producing penicillin by the fermentation method seemed too risky—especially at a time when their industry was already straining to meet the war needs. So Florey's bid for help was turned down again.

Frustrated in his wish to move ahead, Florey turned elsewhere once more. He had been thinking for some time now that he should go to the United States for help. The American government was sympathetic to Britain, and it seemed likely that before long the United States too might be in the war. Maybe drug companies there would be willing to produce the penicillin Florey needed for his human trials. In penicillin there was the promise of saving millions of war wounded. Perhaps the Americans would join his fight against death.

In April, 1941, through a contact in London, Florey communicated with the Rockefeller Foundation in New York City. The Foundation encouraged him to come to the United States. It offered to pay travel expenses for Florey and a colleague to make the trip. Florey discussed the journey and its purpose with Mellanby. Mellanby, who had once criticized Florey for his gratitude to the Americans, now had a change of heart. Mellanby saw that large-scale production of penicillin was not possible in Britain because of the war, and so he urged Florey to take Heatley with him and go to the United States for help.

With wartime security measures in effect and strictly enforced, leaving Britain was not a simple matter. When one had finally submitted all the required forms and answered all the questions, there was yet the enemy to consider. The British Isles were besieged by the German air force, the Luftwaffe. U-boats, the Nazi submarines, threatened the Atlantic sea lanes. The journey Florey and Heatley proposed to take took time to prepare and had to be planned with utmost secrecy. Even Chain, who had approved of the idea, did not know until the day of departure that the trip was on.

Chain and Florey, who had worked earlier in friendly harmony, now had some differences. They disagreed on the necessity of obtaining patents for the penicillin production process the Oxford team had developed. Drug patents were common in Chain's native Germany. A patent would set down in precise words and diagrams the exact techniques and devices the team used to produce penicillin. It would protect, under the law, their exclusive right to use the process. Others would have to pay a fee to Oxford in order to use it. And such fees, Chain argued, could be used to pay for further research. Florey reluctantly went to consult Mellanby and another official on the issue, and, when they disapproved, he dropped the matter. Chain remained angry about this, however, and the relationship between the two partners cooled.

On June 26, 1941, Florey and Heatley quietly slipped away from Oxford. Florey carried a briefcase stuffed with information about penicillin, including copies of *The Lancet* reports and several glass test tubes containing freeze-dried cultures of *Penicillium* mold.

There were no direct transatlantic commercial flights from Britain at that time, and the two men would have to travel first to Portugal, which was neutral. Ethel Florey drove her husband and Heatley to another city in England where they remained overnight. Early next morning, they boarded an airplane and flew to a secret airstrip a distance away. There they boarded yet another aircraft for the trip to Portugal. On landing, a Rockefeller Foundation representative met the two scientists and settled them into a Lisbon hotel.

Lisbon, the capital of Portugal, was a gathering place for refugees from all over Europe during the war. It was also a center for spies. German and British agents operated both openly and in secret here; they bought information, arranged deals, and spread rumors. So Florey cautiously checked his briefcase with its valuable contents into the hotel vault for safekeeping. Each day until they were able to get space on the plane to the United States, Florey checked to see that his cultures were safe. Then the two pale scientists would go out to

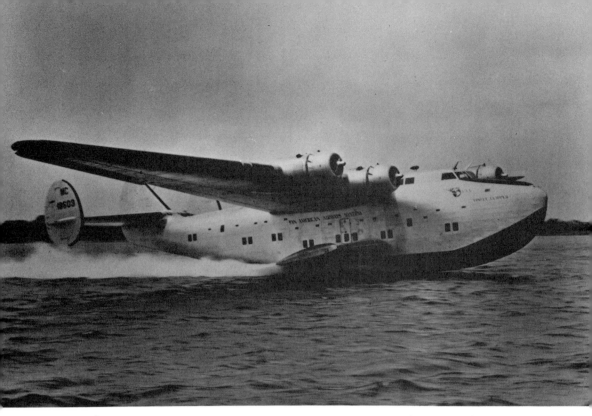

The Pan American Clipper taking to the air. The famous seaplane carried penicillin to the United States with Howard Florey and Norman Heatley in 1941.

enjoy the warm Portuguese summer. On their fourth evening in Lisbon, they finally boarded the Pan American Clipper, the most famous seaplane in commercial aviation, for the twenty-four hour journey to New York.

9

THE FLEMING MYTH

HOWARD Florey and Norman Heatley arrived in the United States on the afternoon of July 2, 1941. New York was sweltering in a heat wave; the temperature was 92° F. American newspapers were filled with photographs and accounts of the newest development in the war in Europe, the German attack on Russia. Less than two weeks earlier, German troops had crossed the Russian border and were advancing rapidly eastward.

But the war news was not uppermost in Florey's mind. He was worried about the effect of the hot, humid weather on his mold. He was troubled also that July 4 was an American holiday, Independence Day. This would mean further delay. So, stopping just long enough to check their bags in a Manhattan hotel, Florey dragged Heatley through the steamy city streets to Rockefeller Center where the offices of the Rockefeller Foundation were located. Though the younger scientist felt, at first, that this hasty visit was unnecessary, Heatley changed his mind as he listened to Florey pour out the entire story of penicillin to Dr. Alan Gregg of the Rockefeller organization. Florey's total commitment to penicillin and his determined effort to save lives inspired Heatley.

Later that day, despite tiredness from the trip, the two men were traveling once more. This time Florey, who must have seemed inexhaustible to Heatley by now, was pulling his colleague along to catch a train to New Haven, Connecticut, to visit his children. Paquita and Charles Florey had been living with Dr. and Mrs. John Fulton for one year. It was a happy reunion. The American physician and his wife, Lucia, graciously put up the two weary scientists for the next four days. These were to be the only restful days Florey was to have in America. During this time, Fulton learned about penicillin and eagerly set about making calls and arrangements for Florey to see people who could help him.

On July 9, Florey and Heatley were off to Beltsville, Maryland, to see Dr. Charles Thom. Thom was the American expert who first correctly identified Fleming's mold from a specimen Raistrick had sent him in 1931. Now, ten years later, the mold had suddenly taken on new importance. Thom arranged for the Oxford scientists to discuss their mission with authorities in Washington, D.C. This, in turn, led to a journey west on July 14 to Peoria, Illinois, to a regional research laboratory of the United States Department of Agriculture where a large division devoted to fermentation research had recently opened. Dr. Robert Coghill, the director of this division, listened with interest to Florey's report on penicillin. It was a presentation Florey would repeat many times before leaving America.

Coghill was impressed with what Florey and Heatley had to say. He was eager to help them and even suggested that a technique used in making beer called "deep fermentation" might improve penicillin production. This method would involve growing the mold submerged in huge tanks instead of on the surface of broth in bottles. But Coghill would need Heatley's help to get started. So they decided that Heatley would remain in Peoria for six months to teach Coghill and his people how to work with penicillin. Florey, meanwhile, would travel throughout America, visiting pharmaceutical companies to try and interest them in producing the drug.

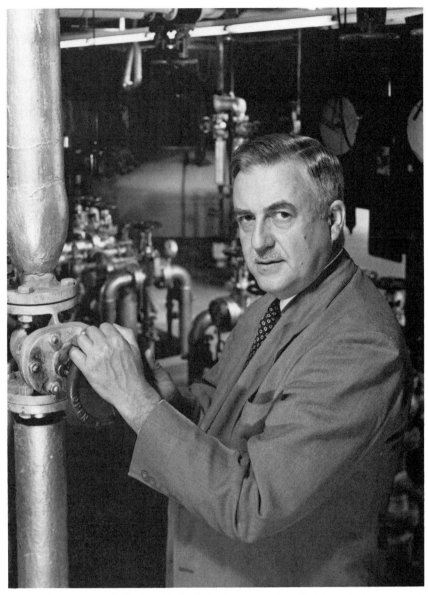

Dr. Robert G. Coghill. As chief of the fermentation division of the research laboratory of the U.S. Department of Agriculture at Peoria, Illinois, he played an important role in the development of penicillin.

In Peoria, Heatley faced two problems. The first was Dr. Andrew Moyer, the biochemist Coghill assigned to work with him. Public opinion about the war in Europe was sharply divided in America at that time. The country had two minds about what to do. President Franklin D. Roosevelt and many of his supporters favored America's intervening in the war. These interventionists wanted the United States to supply military and other aid to Britain and to enter the war against Germany. But a great many Americans, especially in the Middle West where Peoria is located, felt that the country was fortunate to be so isolated, or removed, from this foreign war and should steer clear of it. These isolationists insisted that America remain neutral. Andrew Moyer was an isolationist. And, as luck would have it, he was strongly anti-British. He was also difficult, stubborn, and secretive. It took all of Heatley's good-naturedness for him to get along with Moyer.

The second problem Heatley faced was getting the mold to grow. It seemed, at first, as if Florey's fears that the mold might be damaged in their travels had been justified. But then, after some careful coaxing, the fungus began to flourish and produce its precious yellow droplets. At this point, Moyer made an important contribution. He suggested trying corn steep liquor to boost the mold's yield.

Corn steep liquor was a gooey by-product of the process used to remove starch from corn. It was a bothersome waste material that frequently became moldy before it could be disposed of. And since one of the Peoria station's tasks was to find new commercial uses for corn, such as cereals and other products, the thick messy liquid accumulated, unwanted, in great quantities here. In fact, in no other place in the United States did corn steep liquor exist. What an incredible piece of good luck, then, that the British researchers had come to Peoria! The use of corn steep liquor turned out to be another breakthrough. With other additives, corn steep liquor increased the penicillin yield twelve times.

Coghill's suggestion that deep fermentation could also boost production was tried next. This technique would encourage mold growth throughout the whole volume of a vessel instead of just on the limited surface area. It would permit large drums to be used instead of bottles and trays. But Coghill's deep fermentation technique produced only about half as much penicillin as the British surface culture method. Could there be other strains of penicillia more suited to deep fermentation that might also produce penicillin? The researchers launched a search to find other penicillin-producing molds.

Florey returned to Peoria in August from his travels to drug companies around the United States and was pleased with Heatley's progress. His own efforts, however, had been disappointing. He had visited the eight largest American drug firms without obtaining a definite commitment from any to produce penicillin. Perhaps, in Canada, he would find help. Canada had joined the war on Britain's side, and Florey was hopeful of finding greater interest there. But the leading Canadian company turned him down. The cost, the time it might take to get started, and the possibility that a cheaper chemical means of production might come along discouraged the Canadians from taking on the penicillin project. This rejection in Canada shocked Florey and left him bitter.

Disheartened, but determined to keep trying, Florey returned to the United States. He traveled to Philadelphia to seek the help of Dr. Alfred Newton Richards, the great pharmacologist with whom he had studied sixteen years earlier in his days as a Rockefeller Foundation Fellow. On August 7, 1941, the two men met for dinner.

How often does the fate of an important development rest upon the confidence one person has in another? Professor Richards knew nothing of his former student's work with penicillin, but he remembered Florey as an earnest and talented scientist, and he trusted him.

Richards was sure that America would soon be in the war. German submarines were already attacking American shipping on the high seas. He could see that it was only a matter of time before the United

States would be drawn into the fighting. If this mold drug of Florey's could save lives that would otherwise be lost, then, despite the enormous problems and high cost of producing it, he would exert his influence to help. Richards was Chairman of the Medical Research Committee of the Office of Scientific Research and Development, an important government agency. Pharmaceutical companies would listen to him. The story of penicillin had come to another crucial turn.

Richards promptly contacted four major drug companies. He chose them at Florey's suggestion: among the American manufacturers Florey had visited, these four—Merck Sharp & Dohme, Charles Pfizer & Company, E. R. Squibb & Sons, and Lederle Laboratories—had shown the most interest in penicillin. Richards urged the companies to join the effort to produce the new drug. He stressed that it was in America's interest to do so, and he promised government backing if they would become involved. Richard's support did the trick; he accomplished what Florey alone had been unable to achieve. All four manufacturers agreed to work on the problems of producing penicillin. They would send representatives to a joint meeting with government officials in December, 1941. Meanwhile, one company, Merck, of Rahway, New Jersey, would begin a small-scale project to produce penicillin and promised to send Florey a quantity for his clinical trials.

After three months in the United States, Florey returned to Oxford in September, leaving Heatley behind to continue helping the Americans. Florey was cheered by the promise of a supply of penicillin from Merck. At Oxford, however, he found that penicillin production had come almost to a standstill. The project had suffered in the absence of his strong leadership, a situation he quickly changed.

The promised supply of penicillin that arrived at Oxford from the United States, however, was not what Florey had expected. On December 7, 1941, the Japanese bombed Pearl Harbor in the Hawaiian Islands; this surprise attack destroyed much of America's Pacific Fleet and plunged the United States into war with Japan—and its European allies, Germany and Italy. Merck kept its promise to Florey, but, because of the war, it could only manage to send him a small fraction of the amount for which he had hoped. America now needed penicillin herself for human trials to treat her own war wounded. Heatley, however, managed to ship a drum of corn steep liquor across the Atlantic. And, after seeing its dramatic effect on penicillin production, the Oxford team arranged to get the valuable waste from a Scottish supplier. The extraction plant at Oxford was expanded to handle the increased production. Best of all, a British company began producing penicillin and adding to Florey's supply.

As Florey's stockpile slowly grew, he needed someone to conduct clinical tests once more, someone close to the project who was familiar with penicillin and could be trusted to make careful, systematic, scientific observations. Ethel Florey, who had helped a bit in the first trials, took on this responsibility. She treated cases in civilian and military hospitals. She worked such long hours, in fact, that exhaustion threatened her health. She attended her patients around the clock, carefully measuring and preparing each dose of the scarce drug and recording its effects. Her efforts won her much deserved respect, and the results were impressive.

While these clinical trials were underway, Florey, on August 5, 1942, received a telephone call from Alexander Fleming at St. Mary's Hospital in London. A close, personal friend of Fleming's was gravely ill with streptococcal meningitis and had not improved on sulfa drugs. Could Florey send him enough penicillin to treat his friend? The favor would mean using up all the penicillin Florey had left for Ethel's tests. There was but one bottle remaining at the Dunn School. But Florey could not refuse the mold's discoverer. So he agreed to help on the condition that the case be handled in the same way as the other clinical trials and included in the test series. Fleming readily agreed.

There was no time to lose. So Florey personally took his valuable

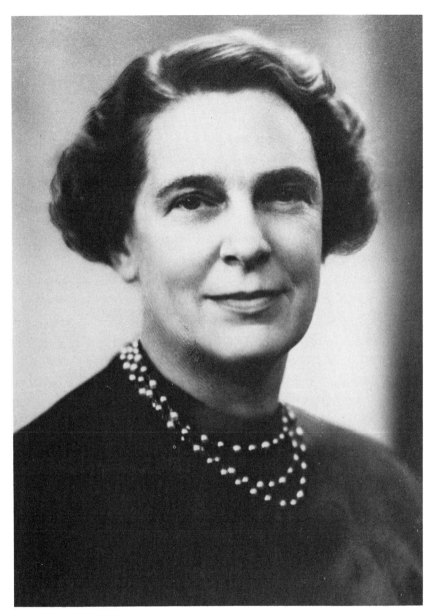

Dr. Ethel Florey, whose contribution to the development of penicillin is immeasurable

drug and boarded the next train to London. He hurried through Paddington Station and walked the short distance along Praed Street to St. Mary's. There he delivered the penicillin to Fleming and instructed him on its use.

Now fate was to play a mischievous role in the penicillin story.

Fleming gave his friend the penicillin for the next six days, injecting it into the muscles as Florey had directed. The patient, however, did not improve. The drug was not reaching the infection in his brain. Worried, Fleming telephoned Florey to ask if the drug had ever been injected directly into the spinal fluid that bathes the brain. Florey had never done this. So he took a fresh batch of penicillin and immediately tried it on a cat. The cat died. Florey quickly called Fleming back to warn him of this result. But Fleming had already gone ahead on his own and injected the drug into his friend's spinal fluid. The patient did not die. He improved rapidly, and word of his remarkable recovery spread.

The Times, an important English newspaper, reported on the development of an unusual new drug from the mold *Penicillium.* This feature article, which did not mention Fleming and only noted in passing the work at Oxford, attracted the attention of Sir Almroth Wright. Now in his eighties, the grand Old Man of immunology who had taken so little interest in chemotherapy could not resist the opportunity to enhance his department. So he wrote a letter that was published in the newspaper, urging that credit be properly given to Dr. Alexander Fleming of his own laboratory for discovering penicillin.

Wright's letter sent reporters scurrying to get a full account of the penicillin story. They thronged to St. Mary's, where Fleming welcomed them. He granted a goodly number of interviews. The modest, white-haired physician with his bow tie and gentle manner looked very much like the reporters' image of the ideal scientist. And so, overnight, the newspapers made Fleming a hero. This irritated a chemistry professor at Oxford, who felt Florey had been unfairly overlooked. He called attention to this in a printed response in *The Times* to Sir Almroth Wright's letter. But reporters who journeyed to Oxford to meet with Florey received a very different reception from the one they'd had at St. Mary's.

Florey was put off by the press. He treated reporters with a minimum of courtesy; he was abrupt and blunt in refusing interviews. On at least one occasion, he even slipped out a back door to avoid them altogether. He feared that the press would divert scientists' attention from their research. And he was concerned that the public would be sadly abused. The demand for the life-saving drug could grow rapidly, and there was not enough penicillin to meet this need. Florey hated the publicity that arose around penicillin and refused to contribute to it. Lacking Florey's story, the reporters featured Fleming all the more.

Fleming's fame continued to grow. Despite the fact that Ethel Florey had quietly carried out 187 other trials on patients, only the one case Fleming treated became widely known. The publicity brought new interest in penicillin. Overlooked in the excitement, however, were Florey's relentless efforts to get penicillin produced, efforts that had already begun to succeed. Kemball-Bishop & Company, a small pharmaceutical firm in a bombed-out section of London, had begun producing the mold juice for Florey, and all at its own expense. The government, too, was beginning to cooperate. It transported some two hundred gallons of the fermentation juice from Kemball-Bishop up to Oxford by lorry.

What an irony, then, that just when Florey's difficult struggle for penicillin was beginning to succeed, who should steal the limelight but the man who had all but abandoned the mold drug, its discoverer. Whereas Florey had been unable to obtain even a hundred pounds through Mellanby to start producing penicillin only three years earlier, Fleming's one successful case and its publicity now prodded government and industry to launch a major effort to produce penicillin on a large scale in Britain.

Thus Fleming, the man who had failed to realize penicillin's potential and had neglected to develop it, now became its leading spokesman. Fleming was identified as the person responsible for giving the world this new wonder drug. And even the early case of the Oxford policeman was erroneously credited to Fleming. Florey was infuriated by these errors and distortions. But Fleming rather enjoyed them and kept a file of the clippings in his office. This collection of false accounts became known as the "Fleming Myth."

Florey finally appealed to Mellanby to step in and correct matters. But Mellanby backed away from the controversy. He believed that the truth would soon come out anyway and refused to become involved. As a result, the Oxford team did not receive its fair share of the credit for penicillin. Florey and Mellanby had misjudged the power of the press.

So penicillin made Fleming, not Florey, famous. It was Fleming who was sought after to speak before audiences as an authority. And it was the aging Scot who put penicillin and chemotherapy before the world.

10

AMERICA JOINS THE RACE

THE race to produce penicillin quickened with the United States' entry into World War II. On December 17, 1941, ten days after the Japanese attack, American government officials met with representatives of the four drug manufacturers that had been studying penicillin. The war, and the first American casualties, created an atmosphere of patriotism and cooperation at the meeting. Here were four large competitive businesses that normally guarded their secrets from each other agreeing to help one another in a common goal—to produce penicillin in quantity as soon as possible. Nothing like this had ever happened before in the drug business. Merck, Pfizer, Squibb, and Lederle would now begin to play an historic role in the penicillin story.

But one remarkable chapter of American involvement, a little known one, had come much earlier. It occurred before the United States was plunged into the war. It took place even before Florey and his group had begun treating their first human patient, the Oxford policeman.

Shortly after the publication in *The Lancet* of the Oxford team's first report on penicillin, in August,

1940, an American physician named Martin H. Dawson obtained a specimen of *Penicillium notatum* from a colleague. Dawson was on the faculty of Columbia University's College of Physicians and Surgeons in New York City. He was excited by the mold's activity against disease germs and began growing the fungus to obtain penicillin. Within five weeks, Dawson had accumulated a bit of the crude drug, and on October 15, 1940, he injected it into a patient dying from an infection of the lining and valves of the heart. This took place four months before Florey and his team had treated the Oxford policeman. Dawson was actually the first physician ever to inject penicillin into a human being.

The treatment failed to save Dawson's patient. However, Dawson believed in penicillin's value. He and some colleagues began to grow penicillin in a mini-factory they created in classrooms at Columbia, much as the British group had done at Oxford. But the crude penicillin they produced was not strong enough to cure any of the four patients suffering from heart infections who received it. Nevertheless, in May, 1941, still convinced that penicillin's worth would yet be proven, Dawson presented his work to colleagues at a medical research conference. Unfortunately, he received no encouragement. As a result, he never published his findings. And Dawson by now was afflicted with a paralyzing nerve disease that interfered with his work. Were it not for this tragic handicap, he might have succeeded in making a significant contribution to the penicillin story. But Dr. Dawson died in 1945, and his pioneering efforts were all but forgotten.

Less than a year after Dawson had filed away his notes on penicillin, however, industrially produced penicillin was to have its first clinical trial in the United States. This occurred in March, 1942. And it came about in a curious way.

Mrs. Ogden Miller, the wife of the athletic director of Yale University in New Haven, Connecticut, lay in a hospital gravely ill with childbed fever. The infection had come after she had miscarried and lost a baby. Anne Miller's doctor had tried sulfa drugs, but these failed to cure the infection and the fevered woman's temperature rose dangerously to 105° F. She was dying. It just happened that Mrs. Miller's physician also treated Dr. John Fulton, with whom Paquita and Charles Florey were temporarily living in New Haven. Could Fulton, who was close to Florey, possibly get some penicillin to try as a last resort to save Mrs. Miller?

Florey, of course, had returned to England by now, but Fulton remembered that Norman Heatley was still in the United States. So he inquired after Heatley and learned that the Englishman had left Peoria and gone to New Jersey to work with Dr. Max Tishler, Merck's able and resourceful research chemist. Tishler was by now deeply committed to penicillin's development and was making important contributions to its production. Through Heatley and Tishler, Fulton hastily obtained consent to release the precious drug.

Mrs. Miller's condition was growing worse hour by hour, and the supply of penicillin was sped to New Haven. It arrived on Saturday morning, March 14—but without any instructions on how to administer it. Desperate phone calls to New Jersey finally persuaded Heatley, who was not a physician and was therefore reluctant to give clinical advice, to tell how the Oxford team had given penicillin in test cases. The drug was injected, and Mrs. Miller began to improve. Within twenty-four hours, her fever disappeared. She continued to get better with regular penicillin treatments and made a complete recovery. American industrially produced penicillin had passed its first test.

An interesting sidelight to this case, one that shows the scarcity of the drug, was that Norman Heatley himself traveled up to New Haven to collect the woman's urine. Undoubtedly he recalled the Oxford policeman who had died only one year earlier for lack of enough penicillin. So Heatley prepared to extract the medicine from the urine to use again.

In the United States, there was only enough penicillin for ten more clinical trials in the next three months. But production steadily increased and, by year's end, 1942, ninety more persons had been treated with the drug. Penicillin had been shown to fight streptococcal and staphylococcal infections, and now researchers were eager to test it against a wide range of disease-causing germs. They wished to learn the best ways of using this miraculous new agent. At the same time, however, people who might be saved by penicillin were dying. Physicians, patients, and relatives of the ill were learning about penicillin and pleading for it.

What more agonizing responsibility could there be than to decide who should receive the scarce, life-saving drug? Dr. Chester Keefer, a distinguished Boston physician, was appointed to head a committee to oversee the distribution and use of penicillin. Despite terrible pressures and heart-rending appeals, Dr. Keefer tried to exercise this authority fairly. When a terrible fire in a Boston nightclub, the Coconut Grove, burned hundreds of people, Keefer released penicillin to treat them. But, in general, patients selected for treatment had to be carefully studied so that every bit of knowledge gained might be used to save others in the future.

In April, 1943, Keefer's committee allotted a quantity of penicillin for the first mass trials on war casualties. A group of men wounded in the Pacific had been taken to an army hospital in Utah. These men had torn bodies with deep wounds and broken bones. All had severe infections that had not responded to sulfa drugs. There was little left to do for them. They were beyond help and without hope—until penicillin was tried. The results provided further dramatic proof of the medicine's value. Almost all the doomed servicemen who received penicillin recovered. Encouraged, other military hospitals soon set up extensive penicillin tests.

By mid-1943, the number of companies producing penicillin had grown from the original four to twenty-four. Even the Canadian firm

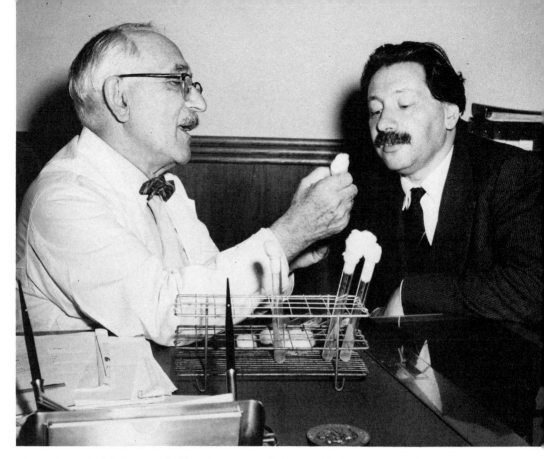

Dr. Selman A. Waksman (left), discoverer of the antibiotic streptomycin, chatting with visitor Ernst Chain at the Rutger's Institute of Microbiology in New Jersey

that had originally refused Florey back in 1941 now began producing penicillin. The supply increased rapidly, but there was still far too little to meet the need. The spirit of cooperation between American drug companies was extended overseas to British firms. Information on improving production was freely exchanged between British and American companies without regard for profit.

By now, too, enterprising firms were beginning to hunt for other promising examples of antibiosis. Perhaps there were more drugs, like penicillin, waiting to be discovered. A scientist named Selman Waksman of Rutgers University in New Brunswick, New Jersey,

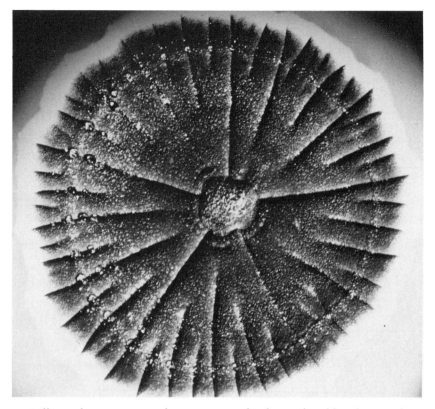

Penicillium chrysogenum. *This symmetrical colony of mold is the type from which most of the world's commercial penicillin is produced. This form of penicillin was discovered on a rotting cantaloupe by "Moldy Mary."*

found a promising agent in soil; he coined the term "antibiotic" to describe such natural antibacterial substances. The antibiotic Waksman discovered, streptomycin, was the first effective medicine for the treatment of tuberculosis.

Meanwhile, researchers at Peoria had continued to seek ways to improve penicillin production. They pressed on to find a different strain of *Penicillium,* one that could grow submerged in tanks and produce higher yields of penicillin. The Army Transport Command

108

was asked to help, and soon army pilots were taking samples of soil from all over the world—from India, Africa, South America, and China—and sending them to Peoria. Here a scientist removed organisms from the soil and tested them for antibiotic activity.

Local molds were investigated also. Residents of Peoria were encouraged to drop off at the laboratory any moldy objects found around their homes. Employees of the research station also joined in the search. One worker, Mary Hunt, was particularly enthusiastic. She picked through garbage cans, trash, and litter in town so often that shopkeepers soon called her "Moldy Mary." But Moldy Mary would not be discouraged.

One day in the summer of 1943, Mary Hunt found a rotting cantaloupe with mold on it that she described as having "a pretty, golden look." She delivered it to the laboratory where it was tested along with all the others that had been collected. This fungus, however, turned out to be exactly the elusive mold that was sought. It grew well submerged and yielded more than twice the amount of penicillin that Fleming's strain produced.

Up until this time, when the cantaloupe strain *(Penicillium chrysogenum)* was introduced, every bit of research on penicillin had come from the original specimen Fleming had rescued from ruin. This probably accounts for two persistent myths. The first is that Fleming's rare strain of *Penicillium* was the only strain to produce the wonder drug. Though it was a stroke of incredible good luck that a penicillin-producing strain found its way into Fleming's petri-dish culture, other strains of this common group of molds also kill germs. The second myth is that Fleming's specimen continues to this day to be the source of all penicillin. In fact, it was dropped from production in 1943.

Moldy Mary's contribution, the cantaloupe strain that would grow submerged, made another breakthrough possible. Charles Pfizer & Company of Brooklyn, New York, a firm that used deep fermen-

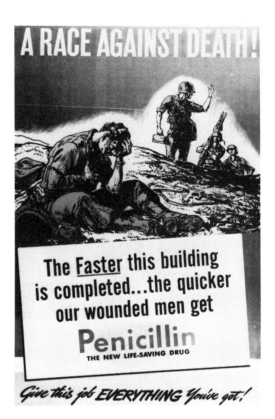

A wartime poster stresses the urgency of producing penicillin.

tation to produce chemicals for the food and beverage industry, took over Peoria's research efforts with the drug. But could a private company risk its money and resources on a large-scale project to produce penicillin by deep fermentation when a cheaper chemical means might come along to make its investment unprofitable?

Pfizer decided to gamble. The possibility of producing penicillin in quantity, when it was so urgently needed, seemed worth the risk. Pfizer's chemical engineers soon devised an ingenious way to improve penicillin production. This method involved blowing sterile, germ-free air into the fermentation tanks in such a way that the contents were stirred continually as they were aerated. This technique resulted in a major increase in penicillin yields. By 1944, Pfizer had a large-scale, deep fermentation plant in operation.

In four years, penicillin production had changed from a bottle and bedpan setup at Oxford to a major facility in Brooklyn with towering tanks that each contained ten thousand gallons of medium. During the first half of 1943, the total production of penicillin in the United States was some 800 million units. In the last six months of 1943, after the discovery of the high-yielding strain, production increased to just over 20 billion units. Pfizer's new fermentation methods in 1944 swelled production eighty times; about 1600 billion units were produced that year. And this amount was multiplied four times more in 1945. As production soared, the price of penicillin fell rapidly. In 1944, the cost of one million units, an average treatment for a mild infection then, was $200, if one could get the drug. The following year, the cost of the same treatment had dropped to $6.50. Mass production eventually dropped the cost still further to about $1.50 and, still later, to pennies.

Of all the American contributions to the penicillin story—corn steep liquor, the high-yielding cantaloupe mold, deep fermentation—the last breakthrough was unquestionably the most important. In 1944, British pharmaceutical companies sent scientists to the United States to learn the deep fermentation method. The British companies, however, had to pay a small licensing fee for its use. Though this charge was considered fair and only a modest return of the American companies' costly investment, it became a source of controversy for a time.

Some claimed that American industry had taken unfair advantage and profited at British expense when the British had brought penicillin over and shared it with the United States. Others argued that though it was discovered and developed in England, penicillin became available as a common, inexpensive medicine for the whole world because of American technology. That the trans-Atlantic partnership between

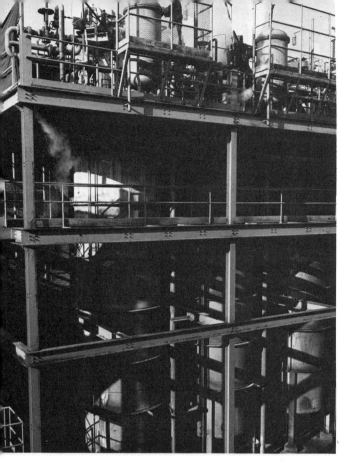

Left: *Penicillin advanced from fermentation in bedpans and bottles at Oxford, England, to large-scale production in the United States. These are the giant fermentation tanks of Merck and Company at Danville, Pennsylvania, 1961.*

Below: *Compounding tanks. Part of the penicillin production process at Pfizer's plant in Brooklyn, New York, about 1966.*

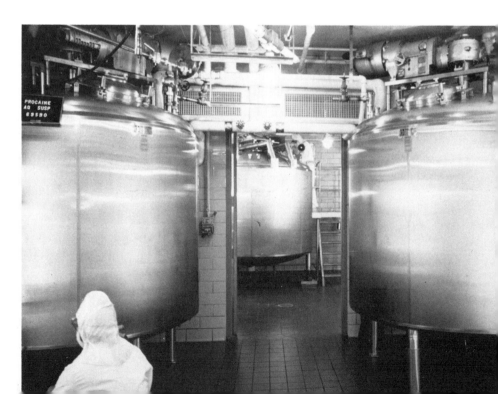

Right: *Here technicians check the strength of samples of penicillin before the drug is packaged for sale, 1948.*

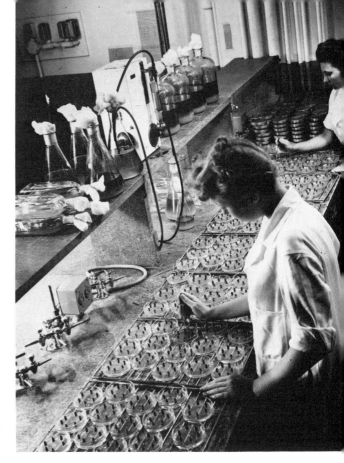

Below: *After the antibiotic vials have been stoppered and sealed, they are inspected and checked again before being shipped.*

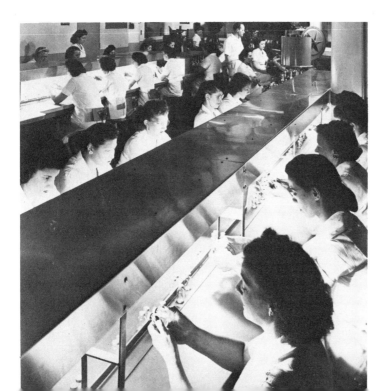

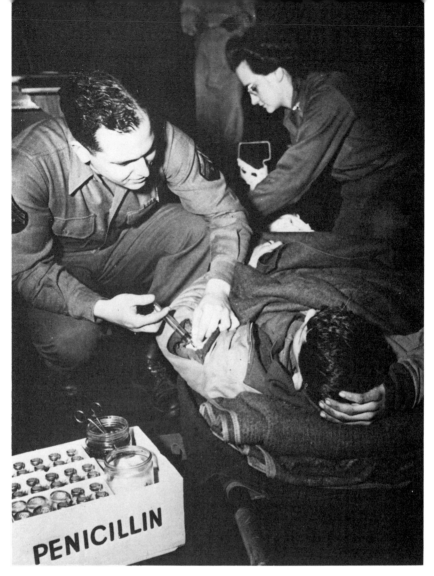

A wounded American soldier receives penicillin as a preventative against infection at a U.S. evacuation hospital in Luxemburg, January 25, 1945.

British and American science was a huge success, however, was beyond question.

Stockpiles of penicillin were gathered in depots in England and were on hand in time for the Allied invasion of France, D-Day, June 6, 1944, the beginning of the drive that would defeat the Nazis and

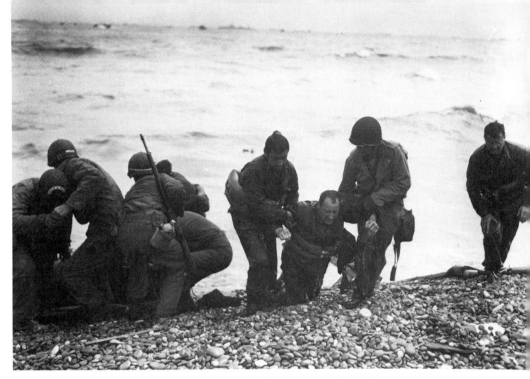

American troops assist wounded buddies on D-Day, June 6, 1944.

American medical corpsmen administer aid to survivor of a landing craft sunk somewhere off the coast of northern France, June, 1944.

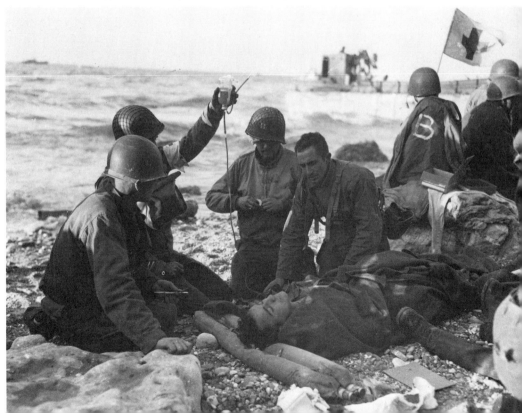

free Europe. Heroes in white coats in laboratories and drug companies contributed to the victory. By the time Germany surrendered, in May of 1945, penicillin had saved millions of lives.

Research had established, meanwhile, that penicillin was effective against the germ that caused syphilis. The antibiotic was safer and easier to take than Paul Ehrlich's Salvarsan, so penicillin quickly replaced it. But Ehrlich's faith had been rewarded, even though it was not his "magic bullet" but penicillin that led the way into the promised age of chemotherapy.

The development of penicillin is history now. The torchbearers—Pasteur, Koch, Ehrlich, Fleming, Florey, and Chain—are all gone. But the light of their torches still glows, and the race continues. The story of penicillin, like all stories of science, has no ending.

EPILOGUE

Penicillin has become the most widely used medicine in the world to fight infectious diseases. Physicians in the United States alone write more than eighty million prescriptions for it each year. Hardly a family exists in the United States, England, and other developed nations that penicillin has not affected. And the wonder drug is being used increasingly in the developing countries as well.

By curing infectious diseases, especially in children, and by sparing the elderly, penicillin has helped substantially to lengthen overall human life expectancy. About forty years before penicillin, the average length of life from birth to death in the United States was less than fifty years. Four decades after penicillin and the other antibiotics it led to, along with advances in immunology, nutrition, and sanitation, the average life-span had increased to more than seventy years.

How safe is penicillin? Some people are dangerously allergic to the drug. These individuals must be treated with other agents. But for most people, penicillin is still remarkably free from harmful side effects and remains one of the safest medicines available. In fact, its safety has led to its overuse and, in turn, to a new problem.

The overuse of penicillin and certain other antibiotics in people and its use as an additive to animal feed to produce healthier, more profitable cattle, pigs, and poultry have led to the development of certain bacteria that resist the antibiotics. This increasingly serious threat worries scientists, who must constantly seek newer, more effective agents against these resistant germs.

Penicillin is a bountiful source from which many new antibacterial agents have arisen. The riddle of penicillin's structure defied some one thousand chemists working in thirty-nine laboratories in the United States and Britain. Then, in 1957, after all others had given up, Dr. John C. Sheehan of the Massachusetts Institute of Technology brought some nine years of persistent effort to a successful end by synthesizing penicillin—making it entirely by laboratory means from chemicals without the mold. Sheehan's triumph opened the door to the development of a host of new medicines based on penicillin's structure, agents able to attack resistant germs.

But penicillin has provided even more. It has brought about new strategies in medical treatment. The antibiotics have extended the range of patients and problems that can be treated surgically. Antibiotics reduce the danger that germs will be spread throughout the body when a patient with an infection needs surgery. So there is less risk, for example, in operating on severely injured people. Fewer arms and legs are being amputated. In fact, severed limbs are now being reattached. And the example of penicillin has been a model for chemotherapy in cancer research. Scientists are seeking agents that will attack cancer cells without harming healthy ones, the way penicillin destroys harmful germs without damaging normal cells.

Penicillin changed the direction of biomedical science. The search for progress through vaccines largely gave way to exciting advances in chemotherapy. But immunology has not stood still. Vaccines for

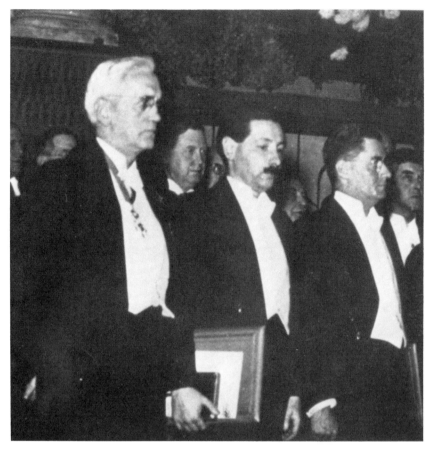

Receiving the Nobel Prize in December, 1945, from the left, Sir Alexander Fleming, Dr. Ernst Chain, and Sir Howard Florey

polio, mumps, measles, and pneumonia have been developed. And Almroth Wright's prophesy that "the doctor of the future will be an immunizer" should not be forgotten. For there is promising research on cancer, multiple sclerosis, and senility that may bear him out.

But what if penicillin were discovered today? Could a would-be Howard Florey ever succeed in getting penicillin through the maze of regulations designed to protect us from harmful drugs? Florey's tiny supply of penicillin would never be sufficient to meet the strict requirements for mass testing that exist today. How can we best balance the needs for safety against the opportunities for making life-saving breakthroughs? Could the penicillin story be repeated?

On December 10, 1945, in recognition of their outstanding contributions, the King of Sweden presented Alexander Fleming, Howard Florey, and Ernst Chain, the torchbearers most responsible for penicillin, with the distinguished Nobel Prize for Medicine.

NOTES

Page 17. *Before antiseptics*. In the 1840s, about twenty years before Lister began to use antiseptics, Ignaz Philipp Semmelweis, a young Hungarian physician, became convinced that doctors with unclean hands caused women in childbirth to become infected with deadly childbed fever. But his colleagues were insulted by the suggestion that they transmitted the disease. Semmelweis knew nothing about germs and failed to persuade his fellow physicians to follow his example and wash before attending their patients. Sadly, Semmelweis died at forty-seven from an infected finger just about the time that Pasteur was discovering the role of germs in causing disease. Had Semmelweis lived a little longer, he might have received the recognition he so deserved.

Page 17. *Lister*. It is interesting to note that Joseph Lister was aware that certain molds stopped the growth of germs and, in fact, wrote to his brother that he planned to use a strain of *Penicillium* (*Penicillium glaucum*) as an antiseptic in surgery. There is evidence that Lister did use this mold as an antiseptic some fifty years before Alexander Fleming's discovery. But Lister never published his results.

Page 19. *Meister*. When Joseph Meister became a man, he worked as gatekeeper at the Pasteur Institute in Paris where Pasteur is buried. When the Germans occupied Paris in World War II, Meister chose to commit suicide rather than personally allow the Nazis to enter the tomb of the man who had saved him.

Page 36. *Harmless germs*. The vast majority of bacteria are harmless and some are even helpful. There are bacteria, for example, living deep within our bodies, in our intestines, that produce substances important to our health. Few kinds of germs cause disease.

Page 65. *Penicillin extraction.* When Heatley used the ether and water method to extract penicillin, he was actually reinventing a process that Dr. L. B. Holt in Fleming's laboratory had developed six years earlier, in 1934. But Heatley knew nothing of Holt's unpublished work.

Pages 66-67. *Animal experiments.* That Florey never experimented with penicillin in guinea pigs was a stroke of luck because the development of penicillin might have stopped right then. The mold drug is safe for most laboratory animals, but it happens to be poisonous to guinea pigs.

Page 71. *Reporting the "miracle."* The member of the Oxford team whom Florey called to share his exciting news that day, May 26, 1940, was Dr. Margaret Jennings. Jennings, a friend and colleague of some thirty years, married Florey in June, 1967, the year after the death of Florey's first wife, Ethel.

Page 75. *Dr. and Mrs. John Fulton.* Lucia Fulton continues to see Paquita and Charles Florey when they return to America with their children to visit her from time to time. John Fulton died in 1960.

Page 104. *Dawson's colleague.* Dr. Roger Reid of Pennsylvania State University provided Dawson with the *Penicillium* mold. As a graduate student in 1933, Reid had obtained a specimen of *P. notatum* from Dr. Charles Thom, the American expert on molds. Reid intended to study the mold for his research project in preparing for his doctoral degree (Ph.D.). But he decided not to go ahead on the advice of his professor, who felt that penicillin was of too little importance.

BIBLIOGRAPHY

Baldry, Peter. *The Battle Against Bacteria*. Cambridge: Cambridge University Press, 1976.

Bickel, Lennard. *Rise Up To Life: A Biography of Howard Walter Florey Who Gave Penicillin to the World*. New York: Charles Scribner's Sons, 1972.

Coghill, Robert D. "Penicillin, Science's Cinderella." *Chemical and Engineering News,* April 25, 1944, p. 588 + .

Colebrook, Leonard. *Almroth Wright*. London: William Heinemann Medical Books, 1954.

Commager, Henry Steele. *The Pocket History of the Second World War*. New York: Pocket Book, 1945.

De Kruif, Paul. *Microbe Hunters*. New York: Harcourt, Brace & World, Inc., 1926, 1953.

Dohrmann, George J. "Dr. John Fulton and Penicillin." *Surgical Neurology,* Vol. 3, No. 5, May 1975, p. 12–15.

Dubos, René. *Louis Pasteur*. New York: Charles Scribner's Sons, 1950, 1976.

Hare, Ronald. *The Birth of Penicillin*. London: George Allen and Unwin Ltd., 1970.

Inglis, Brian. *A History of Medicine*. Cleveland and New York: The World Publishing Company, 1965.

Life's Picture History of World War II. New York: Time Inc., 1950.

Ludovici, L. J. *Fleming, Discoverer of Penicillin*. Indiana: Indiana University Press, 1955.

Macfarlane, Gwyn. *Alexander Fleming: The Man and the Myth*. Cambridge: Harvard University Press, 1984.

123

Macfarlane, Gwyn. *Howard Florey, The Making of a Great Scientist.* Oxford: Oxford University Press, 1980.

Major, Ralph. *A History of Medicine.* Vol. Two, Springfield, Illinois: Charles C. Thomas, 1954.

"Man of Science and of Penicillin—Sir Alexander Fleming talks of his discovery and its future promise." *The New York Times Magazine,* July 29, 1945, p. 14+.

Maurois, André. *The Life of Sir Alexander Fleming.* New York: E. P. Dutton, 1959.

Mayberry, Dean H. "Penicillin Chronology." Northern Regional Research Center, United States Department of Agriculture, (NC-173-80), 1980.

Mines, Samuel. *Pfizer, An Informal History.* New York: Pfizer Inc., 1978.

Murrow, Edward R. *A Reporter Remembers.* Vol. One: "The War Years." Columbia Records, 1939–1946.

"New Penicillins To Fight Microbes Now Resistant." *The New York Times,* March 7, 1959, p. 40+.

"Penicillin Synthesis: Success Is Achieved After Many Efforts Had Failed." *The New York Times,* March 10, 1957, IV, 9:7.

"Penicillin's Unfolding Drama." *The New York Times Magazine,* May 24, 1959, p. 40+.

Ratcliff, J. D. *Yellow Magic, The Story of Penicillin.* New York: Random House, 1945.

Reid, Robert. *Microbes And Men.* New York: Saturday Review Press, 1975.

Richards, A. N. "Production Of Penicillin In The United States." *Nature,* Vol. 201, No. 4918. February 1, 1964.

Sheehan, John C. *The Enchanted Ring, The Untold Story of Penicillin.* Cambridge: The Massachusetts Institute of Technology Press, 1982.

Sokoloff, Boris. *The Story of Penicillin.* Chicago, New York: Ziff-Davis, 1945.

"Synthesis of Penicillin." *The New York Times,* March 31, 1957, IV, 10:2.

"The Mold That Fights for the Life of Man." *The New York Times Magazine,* January 2, 1944, p. 8+.

Vallery, René. *The Life of Pasteur.* London: Constable Finch, 1923.

"Why Penicillin Continues to Grow In Importance." *The New York Times,* February 6, 1979, 111, 1:1.

Wilson, David. *In Search of Penicillin.* New York: Knopf, 1976.

INDEX

ABOUT THE AUTHOR

FRANCINE Jacobs lives in Pleasantville, New York, with her husband, a physician. Her two children, a son and a daughter, are now grown. Mrs. Jacobs is the author of nineteen books, almost all concerned with science. They include *Bermuda Petrel, Cosmic Countdown,* and *Supersaurus.*

"The idea for this book came from my daughter, who was fascinated by a lecture given by a chemistry professor on the development of penicillin," she says. "I was so interested I had to learn more. So I visited Professor Max Tishler at Wesleyan and this exciting project began."